Brown's
EVIDENCE-BASED
NURSING

THE RESEARCH-PRACTICE
CONNECTION

Emily W. Nowak PhD, RN, CNE, CQ

Renee Colsch, PhD, RN, SCRN, CQ

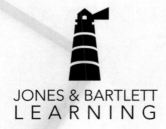

JONES & BARTLETT
LEARNING

World Headquarters
Jones & Bartlett Learning
25 Mall Road
Burlington, MA 01803
978-443-5000
info@jblearning.com
www.jblearning.com

Jones & Bartlett Learning books and products are available through most bookstores and online booksellers. To contact Jones & Bartlett Learning directly, call 800-832-0034, fax 978-443-8000, or visit our website, www.jblearning.com.

27592-6

Vice President, Product Management: Marisa R. Urbano
Vice President, Content Strategy and Implementation: Christine Emerton
Director, Product Management: Matthew Kane
Product Manager: Tina Chen
Director, Content Management: Donna Gridley
Content Strategist: Tess Sackman
Content Coordinator: Samantha Gillespie
Director, Project Management and Content Services: Karen Scott
Manager, Program Management: Kristen Rogers
Project Manager, Navigate: Dan Stone
Project Manager: Belinda Thresher
Digital Project Specialist: Carolyn Dower
Senior Product Marketing Manager: Lindsay White
Content Services Manager: Colleen Lamy
Product Fulfillment Manager: Wendy Kilborn
Composition: S4Carlisle Publishing Services
Project Management: S4Carlisle Publishing Services
Cover Design: Briana Yates
Text Design: Briana Yates
Senior Media Development Editor: Troy Liston
Rights & Permissions Manager: John Rusk
Rights Specialist: Maria Leon Maimone
Cover Image (Title Page, Part Opener, Chapter Opener): © Infografx/Shutterstock
Printing and Binding: Lakeside Harrisonburg

Library of Congress Cataloging-in-Publication Data
Library of Congress Cataloging-in-Publication Data unavailable at time of printing.

LCCN: 2022054047

6048

Printed in the United States of America
27 26 25 24 23   10 9 8 7 6 5 4 3 2 1

Contents

PART 2 Evidence-Based Practice — 169

Lead-In

"Evidence is stronger than argument."
—from *The Celebrity* by Winston Churchill, 1897

Healthcare professionals apply specialized evidence-based knowledge and skills in the interest of patients. This textbook is about the production and use of new knowledge produced by research. As a professional nurse, you should know how new knowledge for practice is produced, how to question the evidence, and how to use that new knowledge in daily clinical practice.

Aims

The first part of this text focuses on how clinical knowledge is produced—from original studies to research literature summaries to the translation of research evidence into practice guidelines. The basics of conducting research are explained so you can understand research articles, research reviews, and evidence-based guidelines published in clinical journals. In the second part of this text, the integration of research into clinical practice settings is examined. This includes locating, appraising, questioning, and translating research evidence into clinical protocols, standards of care, and education.

Features of Note

- ***Emphasis on Acquiring and Appraising Research Evidence for Integrating into Practice*** Part 1 of the text emphasizes how to acquire the best evidence by understanding levels of evidence and how to search reputable sources for study results that are valid. Part 2 of the text, has a strong emphasis on developing skills in appraising the quality and applicability of the various forms of research evidence for integrating new evidence with clinical expertise and patient preferences.
- ***Easy to Read and Follow*** An online reviewer of the fourth edition said this textbook was easy to understand and follow. Following Dr. Brown's efforts for text clarity, we made a considerable effort to structure complex information into a logical progression that is clear and easy to read and follow.
- ***Format*** In Part 1, an analysis and application table is available in the Navigate for you to download and complete as you read each research exemplar. An online and in-text profile and commentary is provided for you to check your answers; this material is presented in a consistent WHY (study purpose)-HOW (methods)-WHAT (results) format to assist you in breaking a research article down into its key parts. In Part 2, you're introduced to a popular evidence-based practice

model–Johns Hopkins Nursing Evidence-Based Practice Model and Guide-lines. The use of this model and associated tools provides context to the content you'll have learned in Part 1.

- *Exemplars* As in previous editions, research articles are used to illustrate the different types of research evidence. A careful reading of these exemplars is essential to understanding how nursing research is conducted and reported. All research exemplars are linked and should also be easily obtained through college, university, and medical center libraries.
- *Escape Room* New to this edition, an online escape room has been added as an instructional activity to promote engagement and active learning. You or your instructor will assign this activity as a summative assessment of Part 1 of this text. You will need to use research evidence to unlock the steps to save your team of nurses from burnout and leaving the profession.
- *Statistics* You will note that there is not a chapter about statistics; instead, specific statistical tests and their interpretations are incorporated into the explanations of results of the exemplar reports. Students have reported that learning about a statistical test in the context of a research study is quite helpful. The index indicates the page(s) on which each statistic is explained.
- *Gender-Inclusive Language* Gender-neutral terms are used throughout the text, and we aimed to provide various exemplar studies to provide a more accurate representation of the world around us and better support all students.

Original author: Sarah Jo Brown, PhD, RN
Emily Nowak, PhD, RN, CNE, CQ
Renee Colsch, PhD, RN, SCRN, CQ

Nursing Research

The knowledge required to understand research articles published in clinical journals is somewhat akin to being a savvy computer user. To be a competent computer user, you do not have to understand binary arithmetic, circuitry, program architecture, or central processing units. You need to know some basic computer language and be familiar with the features of the hardware and software programs you use. Similarly, as a professional nurse in clinical care, you do not need to know all the different ways of obtaining samples, how to choose an appropriate research design, or how to decide on the best statistical test. But you do need to be able to read study reports with a basic understanding of the methods used and what the results mean.

The first part of the text aims to introduce you to research methods and different kinds of research **evidence**. To accomplish this, seven research articles have been chosen as exemplars of each primary research method. Using exemplar articles allows us to explain research methods and results by pointing them out in the context of an actual study. We strongly recommend that you read all the articles in their entirety. Articles are linked within the text and can also be easily accessed using your college, university, or medical library. Admittedly, you might *get what you need by* reading just the abstract. Nevertheless, *if* you really want to acquire the knowledge and skills needed to become a nurse who can read and practice professional health literature, you will have to read the exemplary articles in their entirety. Doing so will help you acquire: (1) an understanding of research methods and results; (2) the ability to extract key information from research reports; and (3) the skill to evaluate whether the research evidence is valid, reliable, and applicable to your practice. The abstract is just a sketch and lacks the details needed to acquire knowledge and skills.

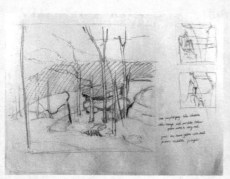 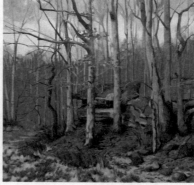

Courtesy of Abby Laux, Landscape Artist of Indiana, U.S.A.

One other advisory: Research and **evidence-based practice** knowledge are built from the simple to the more complex across the text. If you do not master early information, you will struggle when more complex information is presented later in the text. For readers who like to know where their learning will take them, an overview of the text's learning progression is graphically displayed in **Figure P1-1**. The primary learning goals are in the chevrons on the left side. More specific learning issues associated with each goal are shown to the right.

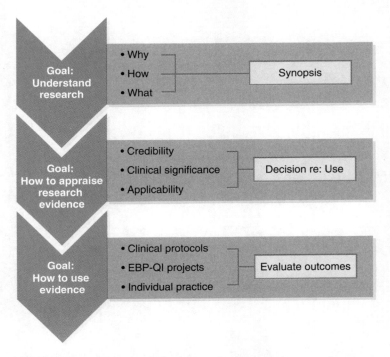

Figure P1-1 Overview of the Text's Learning Progression

CHAPTER 1

The Research-Practice Connection

Effective, safe, and quality nursing practice requires applying scientific knowledge, information, clinical reasoning, judgment, technical expert skills, and the art of compassion and communication to care for the whole person. An essential part of scientific knowledge used in making care decisions is produced by research findings. Ideally, all key decisions about how patients are cared for should be guided by research evidence with clinical expertise and patient values (Dang et al., 2022; Institute of Medicine, 2001). Although this is not a completely attainable goal, large bodies of healthcare research provide considerable guidance for care. This text introduces the basics of how scientific knowledge is produced by conducting research studies in Part 1 and then how to apply that knowledge to nursing practice in Part 2.

Short History of Evidence-Based Nursing Practice

The nursing profession has been conducting scientific research since the 1920s when case studies were first published, and calls for research about nursing practice were first issued in the *American Journal of Nursing*. Now, nursing research is being conducted in countries around the world, and reports of clinical research studies are published in research journals and clinical journals in many languages. In many countries, nursing research is funded by the government, and over 50 countries have doctoral programs in nursing. The growing cadre of nurses with doctoral degrees has propelled both the quantity and quality of clinical nursing research being conducted. In the United States, the National Institute of Nursing Research (www.ninr.nih.gov), a component of the National Institutes of Health, is a major funding source for nursing research. Many other countries have similar organizations.

In the mid-1970s, visionary nurse leaders realized that even though clinical research produced new knowledge indicating which nursing methods were effective and which were not, practicing nurses were not aware of the research. As a result, several projects were started to increase the utilization of research-supported actions by practicing nurses. These projects gathered together the research conducted on issues such as preoperative teaching, constipation in nursing home residents, management of urinary drainage systems, and preventing decubitus ulcers. Studies were critiqued, evidence-based guidelines were developed, and considerable attention was paid to how the guidelines were introduced into nursing departments (Horsley, Crane, & Bingle, 1978; Krueger, Nelson, & Wolanin, 1978). These projects stimulated interest in the use of nursing research in practice throughout the United States; at the same time, nurses in other countries were also coming to the same recognition. By the 1980s and 1990s, many research utilization projects using diverse approaches to making nurses aware of research findings were underway.

During this time, interest in using research findings in practice was also proceeding in medicine. In the United Kingdom, the Cochrane Collaboration at Oxford University was formed in 1992 to produce rigorous research summaries to make it easier for clinicians to learn what various studies found regarding the effectiveness of particular healthcare interventions. At the McMaster Medical School in Montreal, Canada, a faculty group started the evidence-based practice movement. This movement brought to the forefront the responsibility of individual clinicians to seek out the best evidence available when making clinical decisions in everyday practice. The evidence-based practice (EBP) movement in medicine flowed over into nursing and reenergized the use of research by nurses. Three other things were happening in the late 1990s and early 2000s:

- Considerably more clinical nursing research was being conducted.
- The EBP movement was proceeding in a somewhat multidisciplinary way.
- National governments in the United States, the United Kingdom, Canada, and many other countries funded efforts to promote the translation of research into practice.

Today, high-quality **evidence-based clinical practice guidelines** and research summaries are being produced by healthcare organizations worldwide, and nursing staff are increasingly developing clinical protocols based on those guidelines and summaries. Also, individual clinicians are increasingly seeking out the best available evidence to guide the care they provide to patients. The most recent development is an area of research called *implementation research* or **translational research**. These studies examine how to implement evidence-based innovations in various practice settings so that the changes are taken up by direct care providers and become part of routine care. In the remainder of this chapter, we will introduce you to how we can intentionally create connections between research and practice and why that's important to the care we provide.

Research to Practice

In health care, research is conducted to develop, refine, and expand clinical knowledge about a problem to provide insight into the care and promote wellness for persons with illness. The development of clinical knowledge about a clinical problem plays out over time, proceeding from a single study on the problem, to several similar and related studies, to a systematic literature review, to the translation of the systematic literature review into a clinical action or recommendation. Thus, research evidence progresses from knowledge that has limited certainty to greater certainty and from limited usefulness to greater usefulness. As a matter of fact, clinical nursing knowledge is quite variable. Some problems have been examined by only one or two studies, while other problems have been studied and summarized sufficiently so that respected organizations and associations feel comfortable issuing research-based recommendations.

The end users of research evidence are healthcare delivery organizations and individual care providers. The healthcare delivery organization could be nurses on a particular unit or ward of a hospital, a nursing department, a multidisciplinary clinical service line, a home care agency, a long-term care facility, or a rehabilitation team; in short, a group of providers or an organization with a commitment to basing the care they deliver on research evidence.

The use of research evidence by provider groups and organizations often takes the form of clinical **protocols** that are developed using the research evidence available. In contrast, individuals use research evidence in a softer, less prescribed way— meaning that they incorporate it into their practice as a refinement or slight change in how they do something. For example, after reading a research summary about patient education methods for children learning to give themselves insulin, a nurse might alter their teaching approach. Similarly, after reading a study about sleep deprivation in hospitalized adults, a nurse working the night shift might pay more attention to how often patients are being awakened and try to cluster care activities to reduce interruptions of sleep.

Clinical Care Policies, Practice Guidelines, Protocols, and Procedures

Clinical care policies, practice guidelines, protocols, and procedures may all sound alike but they differ in unique ways. **Clinical care policies** dictate an organization's position and values on a given subject. For example, within the acute care setting, patient care policies will outline protocols, guidelines, and procedures on how care should be provided to older adults with hip fractures. **Clinical practice guidelines (CPG)** are criteria that guide or direct care action. Guidelines are developed using clear evidence from the research literature rather than expert opinion alone. For example, the CPG management of hip fractures in older adults provides evidence-based recommendations for venous thromboembolism prophylaxis use in hip fracture patients (American Academy of Orthopaedic Surgeons, 2021). **Clinical care protocols** are standards of care that describe an intervention or set of interventions for a specified population set forth by caregiving organizations with the expectation that providers will deliver care accordingly. A **population** is a group of patients who have the same health condition, problem, or **treatment**. A population can be defined broadly, for example, as persons having surgery; or narrowly, as elderly persons having hip replacement surgery. Some clinical protocols describe a comprehensive plan of care for the specified population; for example, perioperative and postoperative care of elderly persons having hip surgery, whereas others address just one aspect of care, such as body temperature maintenance in the elderly having hip surgery. **Clinical procedures** are even narrower and describe a set of step-by-step instructions of how a policy will be implemented and met. An example might be blood salvage and transfusion during hip surgery. Generally, multidisciplinary groups produce protocols that address many aspects of care, whereas nursing staff members produce protocols that address nurses' clinical issues, such as preventing delirium in ICU patients.

Clinical protocols are disseminated in various formats: standardized plans of care, standard order sets, clinical pathways, care **algorithms**, decision trees. Each type of protocol serves as a guide for clinicians regarding specific actions that should be taken on behalf of patients in the specified population.

Protocols

- Standardized plans of care
- Standard order sets
- Clinical pathways
- Care algorithms
- Decision trees
- Care bundles

Evidence

To produce effective and useful clinical protocols, project teams combine research evidence with other forms of evidence, including:

- Internal quality monitoring data
- Data from national databases
- Expert opinion
- Scientific principles
- Patient/family preferences

There is wide agreement among healthcare providers that research findings are the most trustworthy sources of evidence and that clinical protocols should be based on research evidence to the extent possible. However, when research evidence is not available or does not address all aspects of a clinical problem, other forms of evidence come into play. In recognition that multiple sources of knowledge and information are used to develop clinical protocols, they are commonly called *evidence-based protocols*. Research evidence is an essential ingredient, although, as you will learn, the strength of the research evidence will vary. From here forward, we will use the evidence-based descriptor, often abbreviated evidence-based, to describe protocols and care actions based largely on, but maybe not entirely on research findings.

Evidence-Based Practice

When research findings are used to develop a protocol that is followed in daily practice, everyone involved (patients, healthcare professionals, the caregiving organization, third-party payers, and accrediting agencies) can have confidence that patients are receiving high-quality care. This is true because the recommended actions have been scientifically studied and people with expertise in the field have considered their application. In addition, the consistency of care achieved with standardized evidence-based protocols reduce variability and omissions in care, which enhances the likelihood of improved patient outcomes.

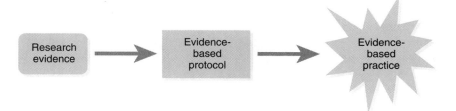

Using Clinical Protocols

In any care setting, care protocols do not exist for every patient population and care situation. Healthcare organizations develop protocols to promote effective clinical management and to reduce variability in the care of their high-volume and high-risk patient groups. If a protocol exists, it should be followed unless there is a good reason for not doing so. Protocols should be adhered to but with attentiveness to how they affect individual patients. Nurses are patient advocates and look out for patients' welfare; this requires that nurses be constantly aware of patients' responses to protocols. If a nurse observes that a protocol is not producing effective results with a patient, a clinical leader should be consulted to help determine whether a different approach to care should be used. A protocol may be evidence-based and work well for most patients; however, it may not be suitable for every patient.

Scenario

Suppose you are providing care to a patient two days after a lumbar spinal fusion, and you observe that they do not seem as comfortable as they should be even though the postoperative protocol is being followed; they have no neurological deficit and the surgeon's notes indicate that there are no signs of complications. You should then ask yourself questions such as, "Why isn't this patient getting good pain relief? Should we get a different pain medication approach? Would applying ice packs to their lower back reduce muscle spasms that could be causing their pain? Is the patient turning in bed and getting up using the proper technique? Should they be sitting less? Should they use their brace more?" The advisable course of action would be to talk with the patient and then with your nurse manager or a clinical leader about how to supplement or change some aspect of their care.

Protocols ≠ Recipes

So, now you know a bit about how research evidence contributes to good patient care. In the rest of Part I of this text, you will walk through the methods used to develop clinical practice knowledge. In later chapters of Part 2, your thinking will turn to evidence-based protocols and to how you as an individual can locate research evidence when there is no protocol for a clinical condition or situation and consider how you might implement the research into practice.

As a Staff Nurse

After being in the staff nurse role for a while, you may be asked to participate in a project to develop or update a care protocol or procedure. Often, your organization will adapt an evidence-based guideline issued by a professional association, leading healthcare system, or government organization. Other times, an evidence-based guideline will not be available, but a research summary relative to the clinical problem will have been published, and its conclusions will be used in developing the protocol. To contribute to a protocol project, you will need to know how to read and understand research articles published in professional nursing journals and on trustworthy healthcare Internet sites.

Scenario

You are working in a pediatric urgent care clinic and are asked to be a member of a workgroup revising the protocol for evaluating and treating children with fever who are suspected of having a urinary tract infection. You may be asked to read, appraise, and report to the group about an evidence-based clinical guideline produced by a leading pediatric hospital. To fulfil this assignment, you should be able to formulate a reasonably informed opinion on the extent to which the guideline recommendations are evidence-based and were produced in a sound manner. If the recommendations are deemed credible, the protocol work group will rely heavily on them while developing their protocol.

In this anecdote, the protocol project team built on the works of others who had produced an evidence-based guideline on the issue. Evidence-based guidelines and protocols may sound similar, but they are different in a significant way. Evidence-based guidelines (1) draw directly on the research evidence, (2) are produced by experts from a variety of work settings, and (3) consist of a set of evidence-based recommendations that are not intended for a particular setting. In contrast, clinical protocols are produced by providers in a healthcare setting for that setting; often, they are translations of an evidence-based guideline that keep the essential nature of the guideline recommendations but tweak them to fit into the routines and resources of the particular setting.

> **Guideline:**
> A set of recommendations for the care of a patient population that is issued by a professional association, leading healthcare center, or government organization. Guidelines are not setting specific.
>
> **Protocol:**
> A set of care actions for a patient population that has been endorsed by the hospital, agency, clinic, or healthcare facility. Protocols are setting-specific.

Your Path to Evidence-Based Practice

We want to emphasize that the point of this text and the course you are taking is not to prepare you to become a nurse researcher but rather to help you be an informed consumer of nursing research, that is, a true professional clinician. In Part 1 you will start by learning about individual studies, then about research summaries, and last about clinical practice guidelines—the three major forms of research evidence. Your goal in reading about them will be to grasp *why* the study/summary/guideline was done, *how* it was done, and *what* was found.

Because this text is a primer, only the most widely used and important types of research are presented. The information provided is selective—it is not a comprehensive reference source regarding research methodology. It does not delve deeply into methodological issues; it does not explain all research designs, methods, and statistics. However, it does provide an introduction to research methods and results that serve as a foundation for judging the credibility of a study/summary/guideline.

In Part 2 you will learn about using research evidence in nursing practice. You will revisit the studies/summaries/guidelines you read in Part 1 to learn how to critically appraise their soundness, and consider their **applicability** to a particular setting. You will also learn about how organizations use research evidence to develop clinical protocols and how to use research evidence in your clinical practice.

You, the Learner

The exploration of evidence-based nursing in this text assumes that you (1) have had an introduction to statistics course; (2) have some experience in clinical settings; and (3) are committed to excellence in your professional practice.

Other Learning Resources

In reading this text, and indeed in your reading of research articles once you have graduated, you may want to have your statistics resources (text, online tools) handy to look up statistical terms and tests you have forgotten or never learned. Your statistics text does not need to be new. Earlier editions are often available very inexpensively, and statistics do not change much from edition to edition. Make sure you use a basic book, not an advanced one written for researchers. If in doubt, ask your faculty for a suggestion.

For a full suite of learning activities and resources, use the access code located in the front of this text to visit the exclusive website: http://go.jblearning.com/brown4e. If you do not have an access code, you can obtain one at the site.

References

American Academy of Orthopaedic Surgeons. (2021, December 3). Venous thromboembolism (VTE) prophylaxis should be used in hip fracture patients. American Academy of Orthopaedic Surgeons Management of Hip Fractures in Older Adults Evidence-Based Clinical Practice Guideline. https://www.orthoguidelines.org/guideline-detail?id=1702&tab=all_guidelines

Dang, D., Dearholt, S., Bissett, K., Ascenzi, J., & Whalen, M. (2022). *Johns Hopkins evidenceevidence-basedased practice for nurses and healthcare professionals: Model and guidelines* (4th ed). Sigma Theta Tau International.

Horsley, J. A., Crane, J., & Bingle, J. D. (1978). Research utilization as an organizational process. *The Journal of Nursing Administration, 8*(7), 4–6. https://doi.org/10.1097/00005110-197807000-00001

Institute of Medicine (US) Committee on Quality of Health Care in America. (2001). *Crossing the quality chasm: A new health system for the 21st century.* National Academies Press. https://doi.org/10.17226/10027.

Krueger, J. C., Nelson, A. H., & Wolanin, M. O. (1978). *Nursing research: Development, collaboration, and utilization.* Aspen.

CHAPTER 2

Research Evidence

The term *research evidence* needs to be defined. Scientific research is the methodical study of phenomena that are part of the reality that humans can observe, detect, or infer; it is conducted to understand what exists and acquire knowledge about how things work. Nursing research is the study of phenomena relevant to the world of nursing practice and can be grouped into five categories (adapted from Kim, 2010). The categories and examples of phenomena within each are:

- **The Client as a Person** (motivation, anxiety, hope, exercise level, and adherence to treatments)
- **The Client's Environment** (social support, financial resources, and peer group values)
- **Nursing Interventions** (risk assessment for skin breakdown, patient teaching, and wound care)
- **Nurse–Patient Relationship and Communication** (person-centered talk, collaborative decision making)
- **The Healthcare System** (access to health care, quality of care, cost)

In brief, nursing phenomena are personal, social, physical, and system realities that exist or occur within the realm with which nursing is concerned.

As a student new to the science of nursing, when mention is made of **research evidence**, you will naturally think of the findings of a scientific study. However, as you proceed through this course, you will come to see that research evidence can take several forms, namely:

- Findings from a single, original study
- Conclusions from a summary of several (or many) original studies
- Research-based recommendations of a clinical practice guideline

Building Knowledge for Practice

A finding of a single original study is the most basic form of research evidence. Most studies produce several findings, but each finding should be considered as a separate piece of evidence because one finding may be well supported by the study, whereas another finding may be on shaky ground. Although a finding from an original study is the basic building block of scientific knowledge, clinical knowledge is more like a structure made up of many different blocks.

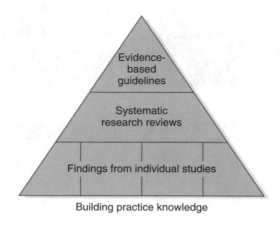

Building practice knowledge

Findings from several/many soundly conducted studies are necessary to build reliable knowledge regarding a clinical issue. Insistence on confirmation of a finding from more than one study ensures that a knowledge claim (or assertion) is not just a fluke unique to one study's patients, setting, or research methods. If a finding is confirmed in several studies, clinicians have confidence in that knowledge because it holds up across diverse settings, research methods, patient participants, and clinician participants.

There are several recognized ways of summarizing findings from two or more studies; as a group, these methods are called *systematic research reviews*, most often shortened to *systematic reviews*. Expert panels may translate the conclusions from systematic reviews into evidence-based recommendations. A group of evidence based recommendations is called an evidence-based clinical practice guideline. Although one could make a case that evidence-based recommendations are technically derivations of research evidence when they are true to the underlying research results, they are considered research evidence for practical purposes. In this chapter, each of these forms of research evidence is introduced briefly in turn. Later in the text, each is considered in depth.

Findings from an Original Study

Most people think of a research study as involving (1) a large number of subjects who are (2) randomly assigned to be in one of several intervention groups; (3) research environments that are tightly controlled; and (4) data that are meticulously obtained and then analyzed using statistics to produce results. Research using these methods is common and valuable; however, it is only one type of scientific study—there are many other kinds. The most common way of thinking about research methods is categorizing them as qualitative and quantitative.

Qualitative Research

Qualitative research can be used to study what it is like to have a specific health problem or healthcare experience. Qualitative research methods are also used to study care settings and patient-provider interactions. The following are examples of phenomena a nurse researcher might study using qualitative methods:

1. The experience of being a differently abled parent or the experience of recovery from a disability as a parent.
2. The interpersonal support dynamics at a social center for persons with chronic mental illness.
3. How members of an intensive care unit (ICU) interact with family members of unconscious patients.
4. How a family makes changes in eating and physical activity over time through participation in a family weight loss program.

These social experiences and situations are typically tangles of issues, forces, perceptions, values, expectations, and aims. They can be understood and sorted out best by methods of inquiry that will get at participants' perceptions, feelings, daily thoughts, beliefs, expectations, and behavior patterns.

Qualitative researchers use the phenomenon they are seeking to understand to determine the research design they will use. Research designs provide a framework or general guide to help answer the research question. The most common research designs used for qualitative research include:

- Phenomenological
- Ethnographic
- Grounded Theory
- Historical
- Case Study
- Action Research

Data collection methods such as in-depth interviewing, extended observation, diary-keeping, and focus groups are commonly used to acquire insights regarding subjective and social realities. Qualitative data are words from what people say, written observational notes of what people do, and other written material such as the diaries mentioned previously. The data are analyzed in ways that preserve the meanings of the stories, opinions, and comments participants offer. The goal of qualitative research is understanding—not counting, measuring, averaging, or quantifying numeric data. We'll touch on qualitative research more in depth in Chapter 4.

Quantitative Research

Quantitative research methods provide a basic understanding of phenomena using numerical measurement. Quantitative researchers use numerical measurements to confirm the level at which phenomena are present and explore the nature of **relationships** among them under various conditions. For instance, the quantitative measurement of body temperature using a degree scale on a thermometer is a precise way of determining body temperature at a point in time and tracking it over time. It also makes possible the study of the relationship between body temperature and blood-alcohol level by 2-axis graphing and statistical analysis. Measurement is also used to test how well a nursing intervention works compared to another intervention by measuring the outcomes achieved by both intervention groups to determine if there is a difference.

Quantitative researchers have specific study questions they want to examine; most often, they involve several phenomena. For example, a researcher whose primary interest is preoperative anxiety may ask a research question on how patients' perceived risk levels for a bad outcome affect anxiety. Perceived risk and preoperative anxiety are the phenomena that make up the research question. However, in research lingo, the phenomena of interest are called *variables* because they are not constants—they exist at more than one level and vary in time, place, person, and context.

> Variables are phenomena that exist at more than one level.

The following are examples of study purposes that could be studied using quantitative research methods:

- The strength of the relationship between health-related phenomena (e.g., between mothers' hours worked outside the home and mothers' level of fatigue).
- Test a hypothesis about the effectiveness of an intervention (e.g., Will a smoking cessation program delivered to small groups of sixth-graders by a school nurse result in a lower level of smoking in 3 years than an interactive computer program delivered and evaluated in the same time frame? The intervention in this study is one variable (it is a variable because it has two forms); the level of smoking at 3 years is the other variable.
- Determine predictors of re-hospitalization (the outcome) within 30 days for persons discharged on newly prescribed anticoagulants. Several predictor variables could be tested, such as type of anticoagulant, frequency of blood level monitoring, age, or lives alone.

Researchers then choose a research design that will produce answers to their questions. A **research design** is a framework or general guide regarding the study structure conducted to answer a specific type of research question. The four quantitative research designs used most often in nursing research are:

1. Descriptive designs
2. Correlation designs
3. Experimental designs
4. **Quasi-experimental** designs (Gray et al., 2017)

After choosing a design that will help them to answer their research questions, the researchers develop a detailed **study plan** that spells out precisely how their study will be conducted—sample size, how participants will be recruited, data to be collected, and statistical analysis that will be done.

Mixed Methods Research

Researchers sometimes use qualitative and quantitative methods in combination with one another; this is called "mixed methods." Using mixed methods may produce a more holistic portrayal of an issue than one method alone can. For instance, researchers used mixed methods to understand child, adolescent, and caregiver mental health problems during the coronavirus pandemic and which interventions were needed. The researchers used quantitative analysis to explore the data generated from the mental health surveys distributed and qualitative analysis to explore the data from caregiver interviews to determine that "COVID-19 and its resulting disruptions to daily life may be linked to a range of MH (mental health) difficulties and needs among children, adolescents, and caregivers in the general population" (Fitzpatrick et al., 2020, p. 1088).

Conclusions of a Systematic Review

Systematic reviews are an important and valuable form of research evidence. A **systematic review** is a research summary that produces conclusions by bringing together and integrating the findings from all available original studies. The process is often referred to as *synthesis* because it involves making a new whole out of the parts. The integration of findings from several or many studies can be done using tables, logical reasoning, and/or with statistics. To reduce bias resulting from the process used to produce the conclusions, the methods used for conducting a systematic review are rigorous and widely agreed upon. The Preferred Reporting Items for Systematic Reviews and Meta-Analyses (PRISMA) provides an evidence-based minimum set of items for reporting systematic reviews (Page et al., 2021).

Systematic reviews, when well done, bring to light trends and nuances regarding the clinical issue that are not evident in the findings of individual studies. We suggest you take a look at an abstract of a systematic review because reading and using the conclusions of systematic reviews is one of the destinations on your learning path, and looking at one will give you a sense of where we are headed. To find a systematic review follow these steps:

1. Go to the CINAHL database on your library's website or go online to PubMed (http://www.ncbi.nlm.nih.gov/pubmed). PubMed is a free, online database of healthcare articles.
2. Type the following text in the search box: "probiotics infantile colic" and click on the *Search* button.
3. Narrow your search to the last 5 years and check systematic review only. That should bring up the citation and abstract for several systematic reviews on probiotics and infantile colic. Locate the review "Probiotics for the Management of Infantile Colic: A Systematic Review" conducted by Simonson et al., 2020. Note that the abstract provides information about how many articles were included in the review, the outcomes that were examined, and the main conclusion of the review. Remember: You are reading a very short synopsis of the review, not the entire report.

From this quick look at the abstract of a systematic review, you should get a sense of the groundwork that has been done by the persons who did this review. In the process of doing the review, they did the following:

- Searched for articles
- Sifted through them for relevant studies
- Extracted information from each study report
- Brought the findings together in a coherent way

This saves clinical nurses a great deal of time when looking for research evidence about a problem they've identified in their practice. You will delve more deeply into systematic reviews in later chapters.

Recommendations of an Evidence-Based Clinical Practice Guideline

The third form of research evidence is the recommendations of an evidence-based clinical practice guideline. A clinical practice guideline consists of a set of recommendations, and when the recommendations are based on research evidence, the entire guideline is referred to as an evidence-based clinical practice guideline. These guidelines are most often developed by organizations with the resources (money, expertise, time) required to produce them. We think it would be informative for you to briefly look at a guideline to get a feel for how the recommendations and supporting research evidence are linked. You will be examining a guideline in more depth in Chapter 10 but to get a glimpse you can follow these steps:

1. Go to the website of the Registered Nurses' Association of Ontario (RNAO; http://www.rnao.org).
2. Click the *Best Practice Guidelines* tab; scroll down to the search box, enter "dyspnea," and click *Search*. The search result will bring up the guideline *Nursing Care of Dyspnea: The 6th Vital Sign in Individuals with Chronic Obstructive Pulmonary Disease*.
3. Double-click to open the page for the guideline.
4. Low on the page under Related File(s), you will see *COPD Summary*. Open that by double-clicking, and you will see a list of recommendations.

The developers of this guideline looked at the research evidence regarding nursing assessment and management of stable, unstable, and acute dyspnea associated with COPD. Based on the evidence, they derived the recommendations listed. (We suggest that you look at the Practice Recommendations [1–5] and ignore the Education Recommendation and Organization & Policy Recommendations that follow.)

The strength of the evidence supporting each recommendation is indicated in the right column, and definitions of those levels are provided at the end of the table; do not get caught up in that right now. To learn more about levels of evidence we encourage you to check out the Johna Hopkins Nursing Evidence-Based Practice tools available free online here:

Dang, D., Dearholt, S., Bissett, K., Ascenzi, J., & Whalen, M. (2022). *Johns Hopkins evidence-based practice for nurses and healthcare professionals: Model and guidelines* (4th ed). Sigma Theta Tau International. https://www.hopkinsmedicine.org/evidence-based-practice/ijhn_2017_ebp.html

In summary, level Ia is very strong research evidence, whereas level IV evidence was obtained from expert opinion evidence (i.e., no research exists, so the consensus of an expert panel was the best available evidence). The evidence levels that support the recommendations are mostly Ia or IV, indicating that considerable research evidence is available for some issues but none for quite a few others.

Remember that you are looking at part of a much larger report. The other document, the complete 166-page guideline (viewable by clicking on *Free Download* tab), presents more specific guidance and a detailed review of the evidence that led to each recommendation. It also informs the reader how the search for

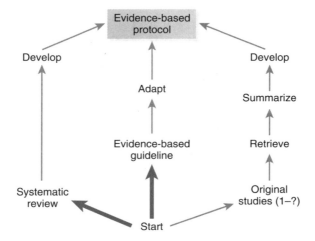

Figure 2-1 Roads to Evidence-Based Protocols

evidence was conducted and how the 2010 update of the original 2005 guideline was done.

As you can see, evidence-based clinical practice guidelines are even more ready to go for use in practice than systematic reviews and more ready to go than tracking down the original research articles and trying to get an overall sense of them. For time-pressed protocol development teams, evidence-based clinical practice guidelines and systematic reviews are the short roads to evidence-based protocols, as portrayed in **Figure 2-1**. Suppose starting the development of a care protocol by retrieving individual research articles is like baking a cake from scratch, and systematic reviews are like using a cake mix. In that case, starting with an evidence-based clinical practice guideline is like buying a cake at the bakery and adding a personalized topping or presentation.

Going Forward

In Chapter 3, you will learn how to read research reports of individual studies. Then, in Chapters 4 through 8, you will be guided through reading exemplary articles reporting five different types of research (one qualitative study and four types of quantitative studies). After that, you will read a systematic review and learn how one type of systematic review is conducted, and then you will read an evidence-based clinical practice guideline and learn how they are produced.

Note that this order is the reverse in which **care design** project teams **search** for research evidence—they first look for evidence-based guidelines and systematic reviews. If they exist and are well done, the team can build on them rather than reinvent the wheel. The order of presentation in this book is reversed because proceeding from original studies to systematic reviews to evidence-based clinical practice guidelines is a more natural learning order.

References

Dang, D., Dearholt, S., Bissett, K., Ascenzi, J., & Whalen, M. (2022). *Johns Hopkins evidence-based practice for nurses and healthcare professionals: Model and guidelines* (4th ed). Sigma Theta Tau International.

Fitzpatrick, O., Carson, A., & Weisz, J. R. (2020). Using mixed methods to identify the primary mental health problems and needs of children, adolescents, and their caregivers during the coronavirus (COVID-19) pandemic. *Child Psychiatry and Human Development, 52*(6), 1082–1093. https://doi.org/10.1007/s10578-020-01089

Gray, J. R., Grove, S. K., & Sutherland, S. (2017). Burns and Grove's *The practice of nursing research: Appraisal, synthesis and generation of evidence* (8th ed.). Elsevier Saunders.

Kim, H. S. (2010). *The nature of theoretical thinking in nursing* (3rd ed.). Springer Publishing.

Page, M., Moher, D., Bossuyt, P. M., Boutron, I., Hoffmann, T. C., Mulrow, C. D., Shamseer, L., Tetzlaff, J. M., Akl, E. A., Brennan, S. E., Chou, R., Glanville, J., Grimshaw, J. M., Hróbjartsson, A., Lalu, M. M., Li, T., Loder, E. W., Mayo-Wilson, E., McDonald, S., . . . McKenzie, J. E. (2021). PRISMA 2020 explanation and elaboration: Updated guidance and exemplars for reporting systematic reviews. *BMJ, 372*, n160. https://doi.org/10.1136/bmj.n160

Simonson, J., Haglund, K., Weber, E., Fial, A., & Hanson, L. (2020). Probiotics for the management of infantile colic: A systematic review. *MCN, the American Journal of Maternal Child Nursing, 46*(2), 88–96. https://doi.org/10.1097/NMC.0000000000000691

CHAPTER 3

Reading Research Articles

To get the most out of a research article, you must be intellectually engaged. One way to be intellectually engaged is to annotate or mark your copy of the article: underline, circle phrases, highlight, or jot comments in the margin—whatever helps you keep track of important information and connect the various parts of the study. When reading a pdf file in Acrobat Reader, you can click "Comment" on the toolbar and use the Comment and Annotation tools. Also, some people prefer to make notes in a file on their computer. You might want to try out a few different approaches; eventually, you'll find what works for you. Below we provide a few tried-and-true suggestions regardless of which approach you start with.

- Create your notes immediately adjacent to the information you may want to quickly reference (e.g., "$N = 54$" for sample size)
- Underline important definitions, outcomes, or findings
- Circle abbreviations that will be used in the report
- Highlight or place a question mark next to statements or information that contradicts earlier statements or do not generally make sense

Over the remainder of this chapter, we make suggestions about how to read reports of individual studies. At this point in your learning, the goals in reading a research article about a study are to identify (1) why the study was done, (2) how it was conducted, and (3) what was found. After you have mastered extracting these aspects of a study, you will add the goals of (4) determining whether the study was soundly conducted, and (5) determining if the study is relevant to the patients to whom your agency or unit provides care.

The emphasis in this chapter and in all of Part 1 is to understand the why, how, and what of a study (goals 1–3). As you read, you may wonder whether the data really showed what the researcher claimed it did or think about the patients to whom the results would and would not apply. However, try to place this thinking about credibility and applicability (goals 4 and 5) on the back burner for now and we'll look at them in Part 2 when we revisit the studies and how to appraise them. You might see a few terms that are unfamiliar to you in this chapter. For now, just look them up in the glossary to get a sense of what they mean, knowing that they will be explained in full as you proceed through the first part of the text.

Goals in Reading a Research Article

- Determine the purpose of the study
- Understand how the study was done
- Understand what was found
- Appraise the credibility of the findings
- Determine if the findings are relevant to the care of your patients

---

Starting Point

Is this a report of an original research study? This seems like it should be an easy question to answer, but sometimes it is not. Some articles read like research articles, but they are other kinds of reports. An article with tables and percentages may make you think you are reading a research study but the article may just be providing numerical data to describe a clinical program. Such data is anecdotal and naturally occurring with no control over its quality or the conditions in which it was collected. As you will learn, it takes more than numerical data to call an evaluation report *research*.

In most cases, the author of a research article will refer to "the study" early in the report, but sometimes you have to read further into an article to determine that it has the essential elements of a study. The essential elements of a research study include:

- Background (problem statement and gaps in knowledge)
- Research question, hypothesis, purpose, or aim
- Systematic methods of data collection
- Data analysis and results
- Discussion of findings (interpreted results)
- Conclusions

If all these elements are present, then the likelihood that you are reading a research study report is very high. Remember that there are different research methods and designs and the essential elements of each type will look quite different. For instance, most quantitative studies address specific research questions or hypotheses, whereas qualitative studies may have a broad aim or purpose. Quantitative studies report results with tables, graphs, and statistics, whereas the data of qualitative studies consist of extended quotes and narrative descriptions. Qualitative studies often have small sample sizes (e.g., $N = 8$); most quantitative nursing studies use moderate sample sizes (e.g., $N = 40–200$). In short, research articles are diverse but should include the essential elements outlined above.

Format of Study Reports

Research reports of original studies are similarly formatted and organized logically. Many journals require using reporting guidelines for main study types. For instance, the EQUATOR (Enhancing the QUAlity and Transparency Of health Research) network aims to promote accuracy and quality in reporting of research. It "is an 'umbrella' organization that brings together researchers, medical journal editors, peer reviewers, developers of reporting guidelines, research funding bodies and other collaborators with a mutual interest in improving the quality of research publications and of research itself" (EQUATOR Network, n.d., para. 1) and is often used as a guideline. This standardization helps you as a reader learn where to expect and later locate various kinds of information about the study. The following is a brief orientation to the primary format of research reports.

Title and Abstract

The title tells the reader what the study is about, including who and what the authors explored. The title is your first clue as to whether the report is likely to be of interest to you. However, titles can be misleading because a phrase or term used in the title may differ from the one used in your practice setting. For example, the research title may state "stroke code" and within your practice setting, it is "stroke alert."

Abstracts almost always precede the main body of the article. An abstract provides a summary of the study, typically in 300 words or less. The section headings used in the abstract are similar but not identical to those used in the full report. The abstract identifies the main points of the study, and after reading it, you should know whether the study is of interest to you.

Let's assume that you decided to read the whole study. Rather than read straight through the first time, you might want to read the introduction and then jump to the discussion section. The discussion summarizes the important findings and places them in the context of findings from earlier studies. Having read the introduction and the discussion, you should have a sense of the study's context and be ready to read the article from start to finish in its entirety.

Introduction

In the introduction of a research study report, the researcher presents a view of the current state of knowledge regarding the problem being investigated; this includes what is known and what the gaps in knowledge are. Study purposes are often outlined in the introduction section. Making note of the purpose is helpful and will be something you will want to refer to later.

Theoretical Framework

In the introduction section of a research study report, a **theory** that has been used to organize thinking about the issue and that serves as a conceptual context for the study may be specified. A theory consists of assumptions, concepts, definitions, and/ or propositions that provide a cohesive, although often tentative, explanation of how a phenomenon in the physical, psychological, or social world works. Propositions are suggested linkages among the theory concepts that have not yet been proven.

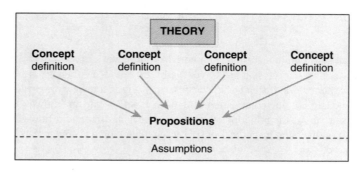

Consider the following illustration to make the preceding paragraph a bit more rooted in the real world. The *Theory of Community Empowerment* developed by Persily and Hildebrandt (2008) provides direction for improving health in communities. Consider two propositions from this theory:

1. Involving lay workers in a community health promotion program will extend access to health promotion opportunities.
2. Access to health promotion information leads to the adoption of healthy behaviors.

Lay workers, access, health promotion opportunities, and *adoption of healthy behaviors* are concepts of the theory.

A researcher conducting a study about improving the health of elders living in their own homes might use the *Theory of Community Empowerment* as a source of ideas for the study. By translating the two theoretical propositions into more concrete terms, the following two study hypotheses are formed:

1. Trained volunteers who collect healthy living questions from elders once a month at the weekly senior lunch and the following week deliver answers increase access to health promotion information.
2. Health promotion information of personal interest will produce changes in health-related behaviors.

As a part of the program, questions that the elders submitted are given to a nurse practitioner who then answers them via video recording which the trained volunteers then show at the next week's lunch. Evaluation of the adoption of new health behavior outcomes can then be measured at 3-month intervals for 1 year to determine if this access to information did in fact change behavior. In this scenario, the theory has served the research by including a component in the trial program that otherwise might not have been included, which provides contextual knowledge for the findings. At the same time, the study acts as a test of the theory because the study has translated the abstract concepts of the theory into concrete realities that can be examined. If the study hypotheses are supported, the theory is supported because the hypotheses represent the theory.

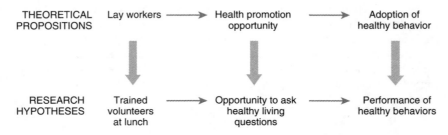

Not all study reports stipulate a theoretical framework; many researchers, particularly those testing physiological hypotheses, do not locate their studies within a theoretical framework; instead, they locate their study in a review of what is known from previously conducted research and what is still a gap in knowledge. More could be said about the relationship between theory and research; however, doing so would be a diversion from the topic of this chapter, which is how research articles are formatted.

Study Purposes

A reason for doing a study may be stated as a purpose statement, aims, objectives, research questions, or as hypotheses that will be tested by the study. Purpose words and phrases you will encounter in nursing study reports include:

- Acquire insights about . . .
- Understand
- Explore
- Examine
- Describe
- Compare
- Examine the relationship/association between . . .
- Predict
- Test the hypothesis that . . .

In the early stages of studying an issue, research is directed at acquiring an understanding of the various aspects of the issue. This can include the problems people with the condition are experiencing, social or psychological forces at work, and what the condition or experience means to individuals. Generally, these early studies use qualitative research methods. The following are study purpose statements from qualitative studies:

- "This study aimed to explore community pharmacists' perceptions regarding their roles, barriers and determinants related to their involvement in optimizing prescribed opioids CNMP" (Alenezi et al., 2022, p. 181).
- "The purpose of this study was to better understand the experiences of maternity care professionals from hospitals participating in a continuous quality improvement collaborative called the obstetrics initiative (OBI) during the early phases of the COVID-19 pandemic in Michigan" (Brown et al., 2022, p. 47).

Note how both purpose statements describe what will be examined but they do not get highly specific about what they are looking for because they want the study participants to highlight the important aspects of their situation and experiences.

After the condition or situation is well understood at the experiential or social process level, subsequent studies may determine the frequency with which it occurs in different populations or measure the degree to which aspects of the condition or situation are present. Later, when several studies have been done and the situation is fairly well mapped, researchers will propose and quantitatively test associations between aspects of the situation or the effectiveness of interventions directed at it.

The following examples illustrate several ways of stating **quantitative research** purpose statements:

- In this article, the authors listed and attempted to answer the following questions regarding the complex relationships between obesity, adipose tissue, and inflammation. Questions included: "Is adipose tissue only made up of adipocytes? Are adipocytes just a reservoir of free fatty acids? Do different types of fatty tissue exist? If so, which types? Can we further subcategorize the types of adipose tissue? Is it possible to form new adipocytes during adulthood? What is the role of inflammation? What is the role of macrophages? Are macrophages central mediators of obesity-induced adipose tissue inflammation and insulin resistance? What causes macrophage infiltration into adipose tissue? What is the role of hypoxia in ATalterations? Is there cross talk between adipocytes and immune cells? What other changes occur in AT in obesity? Does metabolically healthy obesity really exist? Is this a benign condition?" (Guerreiro et al., 2022, p. 1).

- The purpose of this study was "to determine which Nursing Interventions Classification (NIC) interventions studied in digestive stoma patients when they are assessed may best be considered, and to analyze which sociodemographic and clinical factors are associated with these interventions" (Capilla-Díaz et al., 2022, p. 41).
- This study "hypothesized that type 2 MI would be common and would present with distinctly different characteristics and outcomes compared with type 1 MI" (McCarthy et al., 2021, p. 849).
- In a study of the association between Social Determinants of Health (SDoH) and death from cardiovascular disease (CVD) or opioid use, this study sought "to examine the relationship between 1) county-level SDoH and CVD deaths and 2) county-level SDoH and opioid-use deaths, in the US, over a ten-year period (2009–2018)" (Rangachari et al., 2022, p. 236).

Methods

In the methods section, the author describes how the study was conducted, including information about the following:

1. The overall arrangements and logistics of the study
2. The setting or settings in which the study was conducted
3. The institutional review board (IRB) that gave ethical approval to the study
4. How the **sample** was obtained
5. How data were collected
6. Any **measurement instruments** that were used (i.e., scales, questionnaires, physiologic measurements)
7. How the data were analyzed

Each of these steps will be discussed in detail specific to different research designs later. Information about the sample should be sufficient to inform the reader about the likelihood that the sample is a good representation of the **target population** or provide enough profile information about the sample to let readers decide to whom the results would likely apply.

The information about how the data were obtained includes a statement about the organization that gave ethical approval to the study, procedures used to collect data, and descriptions of the measurement instruments used. Reading the methods section of the reports should give you an understanding of the characteristics of the people who were included in the study, the sequence of steps in the study, and the data collected.

Results/Findings

In the results/findings section, a profile of the sample and the results of the data analysis are reported. The profile of the sample lists characteristics of the sample as its composition determines the population to whom the results can be generalized. **Results** are the outcomes of the analyses. In quantitative studies, results are shown in tables, graphs, percentages, frequencies, and statistics. There should be results related to each of the research questions, hypotheses, or aims. To illustrate, consider the following hypothetical statement that might be found in the results section of a quantitative study: "The t-test comparing the functional status scores of those in intervention group A and intervention group B indicated a significant difference (mean A = 8.4; mean B = 6.1; $p = .038$)." This is a result statement; it reports the results of the statistical analysis.

The interpretation of a result is called a finding. A finding for the result statement just given would say something like, "The group who received nursing intervention A had a significantly higher functional level than did the group who received intervention B." Note how the findings statement interprets the statistical result but does not claim anything more than the statistical result indicated. Findings statements are usually with the results and also found in the conclusion section of quantitative study reports.

To illustrate further, consider the results and findings of a hypothetical quantitative study comparing the effects of a new method for osteoporosis prevention education to standard education among high school students. A t-test was used to compare the scores of the two groups on an osteoporosis prevention questionnaire; the result of that test was $t = 1.99, p = .025$. This result indicates that the statistical calculation comparing the scores of the two groups resulted in a t-value of 1.99, which is statistically significant at the $p = .025$ level. The finding was this: The new educational method, on average, produced higher osteoporosis knowledge levels than standard education did, and there is a very low chance that this claim would not hold up in other similar situations. The concept of p-values will be explained in detail in Chapters 6 and 7.

Results → Findings → Discussion → Conclusions

In qualitative research reports, data (observations, quotes) and findings (e.g., themes) are intermingled. Generally, qualitative study reports do not have a results section; rather, they have a findings section in which themes, narrative descriptions, or theoretical statements are presented along with examples of data that led to them. Chapter 4 provides more explanation of the analytical processes used by qualitative researchers.

When you first begin reading research articles, you may tend to skip over the tables and figures. However, paying attention to these tables and figures will allow you to access the nuts and bolts of the results of the study. Authors communicate large amounts of complex information in the tables and figures with a summary of that information in the main text. When examining tables and figures, it is essential to carefully read the titles so you know exactly what you are looking at. Also, the column and row labels within tables are critical to understanding the data provided. Reading tables is a bit like dancing with a new partner—with a bit of practice, you will quickly get good at it.

Discussion and Conclusions

The discussion section within a research report is where study results are interpreted. When a researcher discusses the study results, they relate the study findings to previous studies contextualizing the contribution of the study. For example, a discussion may read like this: "The results of this study are consistent with previous research done with similar subjects. Author (year) reported that using the teach-back method for osteoporosis prevention increased osteoporosis knowledge compared to educational materials alone. Similarly, author and author (year) reported that following a health education session, males scored significantly higher on standard educational tests; however, Author(s) (date) reported the opposite where females scored higher than males following education on health."

The conclusion section is one of the last paragraphs of a research report. In it, the researcher ties together several aspects of the study and offers possible applications of the findings. The researcher will usually open this section by stating the most important findings and placing them in the context of what other studies on the topic or question have found. In discussing the findings, many researchers describe what they think are the clinical implications of the findings. In the conclusion, the authors are allowed some latitude in saying what they think the findings mean. For example, in the osteoporosis education for high school students example just given, the researcher might say, "The findings indicate that a short educational session is effective in increasing high school students' knowledge regarding osteoporosis prevention." This conclusion statement is close to the findings. On the other hand, if the researcher said, "Short educational sessions are an effective way of increasing osteoporosis prevention behaviors in high school students," the findings statement would be beyond the results because the study only measured the outcome of knowledge, not behaviors. In this example the author is adding an assumption to the results, namely, that knowledge produces behavior change and that is a big assumption.

Authors are also expected to consider alternative explanations and limitations for their findings. This would include noting how research methods may have influenced the results, such as "The sample size may have been too small to detect a difference in the treatment groups" or "The fact that a high proportion of patients in the intervention group didn't return for follow-up may have made the outcomes of the intervention group look better than they would have been if post-data had been available from everyone in that group." At the end of this section, the authors usually comment on what they view as the implications of the findings for future research.

References

The references list should include complete information for all citations made in the text. You might find it helpful to mark in the text and in the reference list any articles you want to obtain and read for greater understanding or because they studied

---

Where to look for the Why? How? What?

- Why was the study done—to what purpose?
- Found in Introduction and its subsections; includes Background, Literature Review, Theoretical Framework, Purpose, Hypotheses
- How was the study done?
- Found in Methods and its subsections; includes Design, Setting, Sample, Data Collection, Measuring Instruments, Data Analysis
- What was found?
- Found in Results, Discussion, Conclusions

a population of interest to you, for example, elderly persons living independently in the inner city. A perusal of the reference list can also reveal other current work on the issue, who has researched the issue, and which journals have published research articles about the issue.

Reading Approach

When you first read research reports, they may seem challenging. It's like any new undertaking—at first, it's confusing but the fog lifts quickly, you get the hang of the lingo, the whole picture comes into focus, and the relationships between the parts become clear. Importantly, even seasoned readers of research reports find it necessary to read a research report at least twice. The first time you may only get a general sense of why the study was done, how it was done, and what was found. A second reading usually results in a greatly improved identification of the essential elements of the study.

Wading In

Considering how research reports are organized and having noted some differences between the formats of qualitative and quantitative study reports, it's time to delve into reading one of them. Your instructor may have you choose one or assign one for everyone in the class to read. Alternatively, several studies are listed on this text's website.

The studies in subsequent chapters are considered *exemplars* in that they are typical or representative of a particular type of healthcare research. Most of the exemplar studies were also very well conducted, but they were not chosen because they are perfect models; all studies have warts. Instead, they were chosen because they used a research design that is widely used. We hope you will spend enough time with these studies to acquire a relatively detailed understanding of them.

References

Alenezi, A., Yahyouche, A., & Paudyal, V. (2022). Roles, barriers and behavioral determinants related to community pharmacists' involvement in optimizing opioid therapy for chronic pain: a qualitative study. *International Journal of Clinical Pharmacy, 44*(1), 180–191. https://doi .org/10.1007/s11096-021-01331-1

Brown, J., Moore, K., Keer, E., & Kane Low, L. (2022). A qualitative study focused on maternity care professionals' perspectives on the challenges of providing care during the COVID-19 pandemic. *The Journal of Perinatal & Neonatal Nursing, 36*(1), 46–54. https://doi.org/10.1097 /JPN.0000000000000623

Capilla-Díaz, C., Moya-Muñoz, N., Matas-Terrón, J. M., Pérez-Morente, M. Á., Álvarez-Serrano, M. A., Montoya-Juárez, R., & Hueso-Montoro, C. (2022). Evaluation of interventions in people with digestive stoma through the Nursing Interventions Classification. *International Journal of Nursing Knowledge, 33*(1), 40–48. https://doi.org/10.1111/2047-3095.12328

EQUATOR Network. (n.d.). *Reporting guidelines for main study types.* https://www.equator-network .org/

Guerreiro, V. A., Carvalho, D., & Freitas, P. (2022). Obesity, adipose tissue, and inflammation answered in questions. *Journal of Obesity, 2022*, Article ID 2252516. https://doi.org/10.1155/2022/2252516

McCarthy, C. P., Kolte, D., Kennedy, K. F., Vaduganathan, M., Wasfy, J. H., & Januzzi, J. (2021). Patient characteristics and clinical outcomes of Type 1 versus Type 2 myocardial infarction. *Journal of the American College of Cardiology, 77*(7), 848–857. https://doi.org/10.1016/j.jacc.2020.12.034

Persily, C. A., & Hildebrandt, E. (2008). The theory of community empowerment. In M. J. Smith & P. R. Liehr (Eds.), *Middle range theory for nursing* (2nd ed., pp. 131–144). Springer Publishing.

Rangachari, P., Govindarajan, A., Mehta, R., Seehusen, D., & Rethemeyer, R. K. (2022). The relationship between Social Determinants of Health (SDoH) and death from cardiovascular disease or opioid use in counties across the United States (2009–2018). *BMC Public Health, 22*, Article 236. https://doi.org/10.1186/s12889-022-12653-8

CHAPTER 4

Qualitative Research

Research methods that seek to understand human experiences, perceptions, social processes, and subcultures are referred to as qualitative research. As a group, **qualitative research** methods:

- Recognize that every individual is situated in an unfolding life context—that is, a set of circumstances, experiences, values
- Respect the meanings each individual assigns to what happens to and around them
- Recognize that cultures and subcultures are diverse and have a considerable effect on individuals

Qualitative researchers are of the opinion that a person's experiences, preferences, decisions, and social interactions are not reducible to numbers and categories, they are much too complex for that. They believe that the researcher attempting to understand subjective and social experiences must let the participant's words and accounts lead the researcher to understandings that would remain hidden without open-minded and probing exploration (Aspers & Corte, 2019). Thus, qualitative researchers go into their exploration with as few assumptions as possible to let participants describe their situation and what they think is happening.

Data in qualitative research may take the form of observations with field notes, recordings and transcripts of interviews, diaries, or other documents. The researcher spends considerable time going back and forth through data and field notes to identify important connections. As the researcher gains greater insight into the issue, the questions asked of subsequent study participants may change, or new, potentially informative data sources may be identified (Aspers & Corte, 2019). The researcher works inductively, that is, moving from the details of what was said or observed to a slightly more encompassing phrase or concept, back to the data, and finally to a set of categories, themes, or even to a theory that portrays important aspects of the subjective experience, social process, or culture.

Research Traditions

The term *qualitative research* actually refers to an array of methodologies with diverse aims, data collection methods, and analysis techniques. Several methodological traditions, developed in sociology, anthropology, and psychology, have been adopted by nursing. The three traditional methods that have been used the most in nursing are: (1) **grounded theory research**; (2) **ethnographic research**; and (3) **phenomenological inquiry** (see **Table 4-1**). Nursing researchers use grounded theory methodology to understand the fundamental social processes involved in healthcare situations, such as the communication processes involved in emergency care transports or how families make the decision for a child to have an organ transplant. For example, in a study using grounded theory methodology, the researchers examined the process involved when adults first initiate the use of opioid medicines to treat pain through enrollment in an outpatient medication-assisted treatment program (Wilson et al., 2018). Ten adults were interviewed, recorded, and transcribed in depth.

In the ethnographic research tradition used in nursing, researchers create detailed descriptions of healthcare subcultures, such as chronic renal dialysis units or Alzheimer's disease support groups from an insider perspective. As an example, in a recent ethnographic study researchers aimed to (1) describe the development of integrated services between hospital-based heart failure nursing services and municipally located home care nurses' services and (2) identify the benefits of this collaboration for the development of home care nursing services. Data were collected over 6 years through 102 observations and interviews. Observations and field notes were obtained from steering group meetings designing the services, visits to patients' homes, and educational sessions. Interviews were conducted with the home care nurses, heart failure nurses, and focus group meetings with nurses working in home care nursing (Bjornsdottir et al., 2021).

The phenomenological research tradition is helpful in gaining insight into human experiences, such as living with a severe facial deformity. For example, in a study using phenomenological methodology researchers explored the lived experience of nurses in combatting COVID-19 in Belitung, Indonesia (Gunawan et al., 2021). These methods aim to produce deep, complex, and comprehensive portrayals of their subject matter. Each of these traditions specifies a research process and set of methods and techniques for collecting and analyzing data appropriate to its purposes. These methodologies were developed for building scholarly knowledge about various issues rather than for acquiring helpful knowledge for clinical practice, although the knowledge produced can be quite informative for clinicians. As you can tell from the studies just described and in Table 4-1, conducting studies using these methodologies requires considerable planning, time spent collecting data, and skill in interviewing, observing, and data analysis. However, data analysis and management of coding are greatly aided by software designed specifically for the purpose.

Three other qualitative research traditions are discourse analysis, historical analysis, and case study analysis. Discourse analysis is used to analyze the dynamics and structure of conversations, such as patient-provider dialogue. Historical research examines past events and trends, usually through records, documents, articles, and personal diaries from the past. Case studies are used to comprehensively understand a single case in its real-world context. The case may be an individual in a particular situation, an event, or an organization. Case studies are helpful in gaining knowledge about experiences or happenings that play out over considerable time or occur rarely.

Table 4-1 Qualitative Research Traditions

Methodological Tradition	Common Aim in Nursing Studies	Data Collection Techniques	Data Analysis Techniques
Phenomenological research	Understanding and description of the lived experience of persons with a particular health condition or situation	1. Select persons who are living or have lived the experience. 2. Set aside preconceived ideas. 3. Engage in dialogue with each participant. 4. Explore the person's lifeworld. 5. Assist person to be reflective about their experiences and what they mean to them. 6. Stay in the setting until no new insights are emerging and all issues are understood.	1. Transcribe interviews. 2. Look for segments in the account. 3. Identify significant phrases. 4. Group phrases with common thoughts into themes. 5. Confirm themes with the participants.
Ethnographic research	A rich portrayal of the norms, values, language, roles, and social rules of a health or healthcare culture or subculture	1. Immerse self in the culture/setting, typically for long periods of time. 2. Observe social interactions. 3. Seek out and informally question good informants. 4. Analyze documents. 5. Take detailed notes.	1. Identification of social rules and understandings. 2. Analysis of social networks. 3. Confirmation of interpretations. 4. Produce a coherent account of the culture. 5. Check out description with key informants.

(continues)

Table 4-1 Qualitative Research Traditions

(continued)

Methodological Tradition	Common Aim in Nursing Studies	Data Collection Techniques	Data Analysis Techniques
Grounded theory research	A theory (i.e., a tentative, coherent explanation) about how a social process works, particularly social interaction	1. Gain access to the social setting. 2. Observe social interactions. 3. Identify key informants. 4. Conduct informal interviews. 5. Keep field notes. 6. Identify useful written materials. 7. Interweave data collection and analysis. 8. Stay in the setting until no new insights are emerging and all issues are well understood.	1. Intermix data collection and analysis. 2. Name what is happening in the data with codes. 3. Analyze the use of language. 4. Proceed from concrete codes to theoretical ones. 5. Constantly compare new data with previously acquired data. 6. Generate core concepts and hypotheses and check them out with participants.

Qualitative Description

In the clinical fields, the knowledge that is more focused and straightforward than that produced by traditional methodologies is often quite valuable. For instance, clinicians could interact more sensitively with teenagers who have been told that they are going to have to have hemodialysis while they wait for a kidney transplant if they knew what these young people think about during the interval after learning of the necessity of the dialysis and up to starting it. A study that focuses on just that issue could be designed by interviewing them shortly after they start dialysis. They would be asked what thoughts were going through their heads, what worried them the most, how they handled their worries, and what helped them during the time prior to starting dialysis. No attempt would be made to understand how the bigger picture of their lives, their philosophical approach to life, social support, or medical history shaped different responses during that time. Typically, no observations of them would be made during that time, and no attempt to interview parents or care providers would be made. The knowledge produced would not be complex, but it could provide valuable insights for clinicians who give care to these young people.

Goals
Qualitative description

The methodology of qualitative description produces straightforward descriptions of a group's perceptions, thoughts, worries, attitudes, and coping methods (Tenny et al., 2021). The goal of qualitative description is to capture the important elements of an experience or situation and produce a descriptive summary. The researchers stay close to their data and to the surface of words and events to preserve the everyday language of what participants said and impose a minimum of conjecture about what the participant meant (Tenny et al., 2021).

Methods

Commonly used methods of qualitative description include, but are not limited to the following:

1. Sampling of sources for depth and breadth of information
2. Data collection by informal or semi-structured interviews of individuals or focus groups
3. Data analysis by **qualitative content or thematic analysis**
4. Findings rendered in the form of categories, themes, or patterns that capture what the study participants said (Tenny et al., 2021)

Purposive sampling can have one of several objectives; most commonly, a sample selection is based on the researcher's rationale in terms of being either diverse representation, demographic characteristics proportionally represented, or the most informative (Tenny et al., 2021).

If you think about it, you will realize that interviews and focus groups produce abundant data, pages and pages of interviews or focus group discussion transcripts. To extract meaning from all this raw data, researchers use a technique called *content thematic analysis*. There are quite a few types of content analysis, and they are quite diverse in purpose and methods. However, conventional content thematic analysis, which aims to produce a descriptive summary of an experience or situation of interest, is the most common type used in nursing studies so this is the only technique described here.

Most commonly, researchers identify small sections of data that convey an idea and assign it a word or phrase code that captures its essence. The code should be data derived, that is, closely representing what was said (Tenny et al., 2021). In assigning a code to a section of transcribed narrative or a section of a diary, the researcher is always aware that an interpretation is being made and, therefore, must be careful that the code does not change the original meaning of what was said.

Content thematic analysis is not a linear process. Instead, it is dynamic and reflexive. If none of the previously used codes captures the meaning of a section of the text, the researcher will create a new code. The new code may or may not lead the researcher to revise the coding of already coded text. At some point, several closely related codes may be combined into one. Thus, there is quite a bit of back-and-forth in the data and an emerging feel for what participants said across all interviews or observations. Fortunately, software programs are available to search through the data, identify and track words and codes, and apply new codes, thereby assisting the researcher in moving around in the data and evolving categories, patterns, and themes.

A list of codes can be informative, but it may be more useful if coding is taken a step further. By identifying similarities in the codes, it may be possible to group similar codes without losing the meaning of the first round of codes. This broader or more abstract grouping may be a category, a chronological order, or a theme. Again, the researcher is on guard to not lose the meaning of the original data and codes. To illustrate, a study was conducted to explore, clarify, and better understand the ways that intersectional identity can impact the lived experiences for Black Deaf women on a predominately White, male, and hearing college campus (Chapple et al., 2021). Data were collected through campus observations, focus groups, and 25 individual in-depth interviews and analyzed using a critical race–grounded theory method. Sections of what participants said were coded as: *hearing and White Deaf people, the burden of being Black Deaf among a group of Black hearing students on campus vs. being Black and Deaf among a group of White Deaf students on campus, and hearing male professors and students in the classroom.* Those codes were then combined to the slightly more abstract categories of *identity is intersectional, the lived experiences of Black Deaf women on campus, and the role of intersectional racism, ableism, and sexism on campus.* Then, following a discussion of the themes, Black Deaf feminism was introduced as a theory and conceptual framework for Black Deaf women's research and practice (Chapple, 2019; Chapple et al., 2021).

Original quote → Code
Several similar quotes → Code modification
Several similar codes → Category or Theme

In summary, qualitative description is a pragmatic approach to qualitative research. It is characterized by using a combination of techniques that produces a valuable description of the experience, perceptions, or events of interest. Any interpretation produced should not be far removed in meaning from the data provided by the study participants. Lastly, note that qualitative description is perhaps the most frequently used qualitative method in published nursing studies.

Uniqueness of Qualitative Studies

Findings from qualitative research often are helpful in their own right, and others produce questions and hypotheses that require further study using more in-depth qualitative methods or quantitative methods. Indeed, many study descriptions of patients' experiences of illness and health care provide insights that are directly useful to nurses in understanding what their patients are experiencing and in communicating sensitively with them. They may also be useful in developing nursing assessment guides and teaching plans. When a qualitative study uncovers or alludes to an issue but doesn't fully explore it, it may be valuable to do a more in-depth qualitative study or a quantitative study. A qualitative study could produce a deeper understanding of the situation's dynamics, whereas a quantitative study could test hypotheses on possible causal relationships or quantify the prevalence of perceptions and attitudes in a population.

At first, qualitative research methods may seem unscientific. Although they are indeed very different from what most people view as scientific, the reality is that these methods have been developed to acquire insights into subjective experiences and social processes recognizing that complex human realities cannot be broken apart, manipulated or examined the way physical realities can be. The rich and nuanced understandings of human experiences and social interaction produced by qualitative methods cannot be achieved using methods that reduce human characteristics to numbers and the context of human lives to the status of variables.

Qualitative studies are sometimes criticized for having small sample sizes or for not being objective. These criticisms are based on a lack of understanding of what qualitative studies aim to produce and how their methods produce unique and valuable forms of knowledge for clinical practice. Both qualitative and quantitative research methods have a place in the scientific toolbox of the clinical professions. Just as a house cannot be built with only one type of tool, for example, hammers, it is that producing the full range of knowledge required for clinical practice requires the use of both qualitative and quantitative research methods.

Exemplar Analysis and Application Activity

Reading Tips

Before reading the exemplar, please note that the structure of this chapter is the same structure used in the rest of the chapters in Part 1 of this text.

Each chapter is made up of three sections:

1. Introductory information about the featured research method in an opening section, such as what you have just read about qualitative methods.
2. A link to the online analysis and application table and a link to the exemplar article in which the featured method was used.
3. A link to the profile and commentary on the exemplar article.

Again, we would stress that reading just the abstract will not help deepen your knowledge about qualitative research methods and the meaning of the findings. For this study, the conclusions in the abstract do not come close to the fascinating, more fine-grained insights described in the Results section of the article. Similarly, the Profile & Commentary section will only make sense if you have the exemplar article and your completed table in front of you and refer to it.

Exemplar

Qualitative Exemplar Article

Semple, C. J., McCaughan, E., Beck, E. R., & Hanna, J. R. (2021). "Living in parallel worlds" – bereaved parents' experience of family life when a parent with dependent children is at end of life from cancer: A qualitative study. *Palliative Medicine, 35*(5), 933–942. https://doi.org/10.1177/02692163211001719. This article is published under a CC-BY Creative Common License https://creativecommons.org/licenses/by/4.0

Qualitative Analysis and Application Table

		Page
Study Purpose (Why)		
Methods (How)		
Design		
Sample		
Data Collection		
Data Analysis		
Ethics Review		
Results (What)		

Qualitative Profile and Commentary on the Exemplar Article

Semple, C. J., McCaughan, E., Beck, E. R., & Hanna, J. R. (2021). "Living in parallel worlds" – bereaved parents' experience of family life when a parent with dependent children is at end of life from cancer: A qualitative study. *Palliative Medicine, 35*(5), 933–942. https://doi.org/10.1177/02692163211001719. This article is published under a CC-BY Creative Common License https://creativecommons.org/licenses/by/4.0

		Page
Study Purpose (Why)	The clearest statement of the exemplar study's purpose is in the abstract under aim: "To explore bereaved parents' experience and needs for families when a parent is at end of life from cancer with dependent children."	p. 933
	They expand on the study aims in the text "to better understand how and when family-centred cancer care can be best facilitated and provided, there is a need to gain an improved understanding of parents' needs and how they managed the end of life experience with their children."	p. 934
	Then under aims and objectives, they clearly state, "this study aims to explore the experience and needs of parents with dependent children, when their mum or dad is at end of life from cancer." Then they further state the objectives "Through the lens of bereaved parents, the objectives of the study are to explore how parents: 1. perceived they managed family life, 2. communicated with their children, 3. prepared their children for the death of mum or dad, 4. could be best supported as they managed family life."	p. 934
	It is important to note that the authors define the end of life, "for the purpose of this study, end of life is when a person is expected to die from cancer within twelve months." And they list the complex challenges faced by parents "reduced availability for parenting; changes to parental roles; heightened distress as they prepare children for parental death; and, or financial implications."	p. 934

(continues)

		Page
Methods (How)		
Design	This study is described as "a qualitative design using semi-structured interviews" and has all the characteristics of the qualitative description: ■ A fairly narrow purpose ■ Data collection from interviews using questions that elicited laypersons' perceptions, preferences, and suggestions ■ Analysis of transcript data using a technique that went back and forth between data and assigned categories, i.e., codes ■ Offered themes that are close to what participants said ■ Produced knowledge that is useful for clinical practice	p. 934
Sample	"Convenience sampling aimed at identifying participants from the general public, a family support service and hospice throughout Northern Ireland (NI), UK." Furthermore, "volunteer sampling techniques were used to assist accrual and representation of hard-to-reach families beyond support groups and hospice services. "	p. 934
	The participant eligibility criteria for study inclusion are presented in **Table 1**.	p. 935
Data Collection	The way that the interviews were conducted is well described. The interview topic questions are presented in **Table 2**, from which open-ended questions were created. The topics started broad and then posed "additional follow-up questions." The additional questions help identify aspects that can place observations in real terms, validating their impression and providing more insights. Data collection was concluded when no further categories were identified.	p. 935
Data Analysis	The table of sample characteristics informs the reader of the extent to which diversity was achieved. The data analysis method was described as "thematic analysis." Of importance is that all authors read the transcripts, and the 1st and 4th authors spent considerable time muddling around in the data and refining themes to capture the data richly.	p. 935

		Page
Ethics Review	This study, as every study, should clearly state ethical approval. This study stated "ethical approvals were obtained at institutional and national levels." A complete discussion of institutional review board review is in Chapter 5.	p. 935
Results (What)	The four themes, eight sub-themes, and **Figure 1**, "End of life continuum when a mum or dad with dependent children is dying from cancer," derived from analysis of the interview transcripts, are valuable and practical. Sufficient participant quotes are provided to reassure the reader that the themes emerged from what the participants said. Many of the participants' quotes are quite powerful in and of themselves. The themes are valuable reminders that parents are often "living in parallel worlds throughout the end of life period, which appeared to impact their readiness to prepare their children for the impending death of the ill-parent." The results at the direct quote level, category level, and theme level are clinically informative.	pp.936–940
	The discussion and recommendations are an excellent summary of bereaved parents' experience of family life when a parent with dependent children is at end of life from cancer, and locates the findings in the context of prior studies on the topic.	p. 939
	The limitations discussion reminds the reader that "Bereaved parents included in this study represent those from two-parent or 'significant adult' families. It is unclear how single parents and those with complex family set-ups navigate this end-of-life experience, despite efforts to gain broader representation by public advert."	p. 940

References

Aspers, P., & Corte, U. (2019). What is qualitative in qualitative research. *Qualitative Sociology, 42*(2), 139–160. https://doi.org/10.1007/s11133-019-9413-7

Bjornsdottir, K., Ketilsdottir, A., Gudnadottir, M., Kristinsdottir, I. V., & Ingadottir, B. (2021). Integration of nursing services provided to patients with heart failure living at home: A longitudinal ethnographic study. *Journal of Clinical Nursing, 30*(7–8), 1120–1131. https://doi.org/10.1111/jocn.15658

Chapple, R. L. (2019). Towards a theory of Black Deaf feminism. The quiet invisibility of a population. *Affilia: Journal of Women and Social Work, 34*(2), 186–198. https://doi.org/10.1177/0886109918818080

Chapple, R. L., Bridwell, B. A., & Gray, K. L. (2021). Exploring intersectional identity in Black Deaf women: The complexity of the lived experience in college. *Affilia, 36*(4), 571–592. https://doi .org/10.1177/0886109920985769

Gunawan, J., Aungsuroch, Y., Marzilli, C., Fisher, M. L., Nazliansyah, & Sukarna, A. (2021). A phenomenological study of the lived experience of nurses in the battle of COVID-19. *Nursing Outlook, 69*(4), 652–659. https://doi.org/10.1016/j.outlook.2021.01.020

Semple, C. J., McCaughan, E., Beck, E. R., & Hanna, J. R. (2021). "Living in parallel worlds" – bereaved parents' experience of family life when a parent with dependent children is at end of life from cancer: A qualitative study. *Palliative Medicine, 35*(5), 933–942. https://doi .org/10.1177/02692163211001719

Tenny, S., Brannan, G. D., Brannan, J. M., et al. (2021). *Qualitative study*. In StatPearls [Internet]. StatPearls Publishing. https://www.ncbi.nlm.nih.gov/books/NBK470395/

Wilson, M., Shaw, M. R., & Roberts, M. L. A. (2018). Opioid initiation to substance use treatment: "They just want to feel normal." *Nursing Research (New York), 67*(5), 369–378. https://doi .org/10.1097/NNR.0000000000000298

CHAPTER 5

Quantitative Descriptive Research

Quantitative researchers approach scientific inquiry very differently from qualitative researchers. While qualitative researchers seek to understand the meaning of human experiences and social interaction, quantitative researchers aim to determine the world's characteristics, variability, and connections. Quantitative researchers measure and count phenomena, then analyze the numbers to portray and determine their relationship with other phenomena. Quantitative research is not a research method; rather, it is a collection of quite a few methods that have in common collection and analysis of numerical data. In this chapter and the following three chapters, the quantitative research methods most widely used in nursing research will be explained.

Methods

A helpful early step when building knowledge about patients' wellness behaviors, illnesses, or caregiving situations is to learn about the frequency of occurrence of the phenomena of interest and the elements and features that comprise them. In quantitative descriptive research (from now on, just called *descriptive research*), data are obtained under natural conditions, with no attempt to manipulate the situation in any way—no treatment or intervention is given. For this reason, descriptive studies are classified as nonexperimental or observational designs. The aim is to capture naturally occurring features of the phenomenon being studied.

To create detailed descriptions of phenomena, researchers with descriptive aims collect numerical or categorical data, which could consist of any of the following:

- Measurements of physiologic states that produce a number value, for example, heart beats/minute
- Questionnaires with choice answers that can be scored, for example, always (2), sometimes (1), never (0)
- Observations that are categorized and/or counted, for example, readmitted within 30 days/readmitted between 31 and 60 days/not readmitted; distance walked in 6 minutes

Some quantitative data are obtained directly in numerical form (e.g., white blood cell count), whereas other quantitative data are produced by converting occurrences or behaviors from their natural form to categories or numerical values. For example, exercise behaviors described by patients can be converted into levels of exercise by the data collector using precise definitions.

After the data are collected, they are summarized to produce a rather detailed composite picture of the phenomenon. The summary statistics used in descriptive research include counts, percentages, means, medians, ranges, and standard deviations. These descriptive statistics may be reported in tables, text, or picture summaries, including line and bar graphs, frequency distributions, and box plots. (These reporting techniques should be known to you from your statistics course.) The composite pictures often portray proportions and dispersion of the phenomena in the population and/or subpopulations, the different levels at which the phenomena is present, and which of its elements or features are most commonly present.

To get more real world: a descriptive study examined the phenomenon of health-related quality-of-life in persons living with a urostomy, which is a diversion of urine to a stoma and bag (Pazar, Yava, & Basal, 2015). Data were collected via mailed questionnaires from 24 patients 4 months after their urostomy surgery. A 30-item quality-of-life questionnaire measured three aspects of quality of life: general wellness, daily function, and undesirable symptoms. In another questionnaire, associated issues including work status, feelings about changes in bodily appearance, sexual life, concerns about odor, and psychological health were scored as yes-no answers. The quality-of-life data was summarized by calculating the mean score and standard deviations for the total questionnaire and each of the three sub-aspects. The associated issues were summarized as percentages of patients who indicated the issue was a problem for them. The findings included the following:

1. In all three areas of health-related quality of life, persons with urostomies had lower mean scores than the population-based norms.
2. Most respondents stated that their urostomy affected their dressing habits (83.4%), sleep patterns (91.7%), family life (91.7%), participation in social activities (91.7%), and occupation (75.0%).
3. Although 41% of the patients worked outside their homes before urostomy surgery, the proportion of patients employed following surgery decreased significantly to 4%.

Study Variables

In the most basic form of descriptive research, one main variable of interest (i.e., the phenomenon of interest) is measured, sometimes using several different **instruments** that assign values to various aspects of it. In addition, several other contextual variables may also be examined. In the study just described, the phenomenon/variable of major interest was quality of life in persons with a urostomy. Sleep patterns, family life, social activities, dressing ability, and sexual activity were some aspects of quality of life that were measured. The contextual variables of age, time since surgery, demographic information, body image, and employment status before and after surgery were also of interest and quantified, even if just as yes/no.

By definition, a **variable** changes in the amount, size, or level within a person over time, from person to person, and from situation to situation. In other words, it is not constant. Most characteristics of human nature and situations vary. Examples of variables are anxiety level, blood pressure, gender, weight, pressure ulcer rate, length of breastfeeding, attitudes toward birth control, family unity, and frequency of hand washing; quite a diverse list. To take just one, a person's level of anxiety varies over time depending on what is happening to them, and not every person on the day of surgery has the same level of anxiety. Thus, anxiety varies across time in a person and across persons—it is a variable. *Home delivery* or *hospital delivery* is an example of a variable with just two variations, whereas *ethnic identification* could have several categorical variations (Asian American, Black, Hispanic or Latino, white or Caucasian, and so on).

Measurement of Variables

In physiological studies, measurement is often made with a device:

- An adhesive pad with an embedded thermoelectric transducer attached to a transmitter measures body temperature continuously.
- A lab test measures serum 25-hydroxyvitamin D level.
- Blood flow to organs and extremities can be quantified with a probe and Doppler ultrasound flowmeter.

Alternatively, a measurement can be determined by an observer:

- Delirium can be quantified in the emergency department using a validated AWOL score from a delirium prediction scale (LaHue & Douglas, 2022).
- Cervical dilation during pregnancy and labor can be assigned a centimeter value by determining how many fingers slip into the opening cervix.
- A pitting edema grading scale assigns a numerical value to the degree of edema observed based on the depth of pitting (1+, 2+, 3+, 4+).

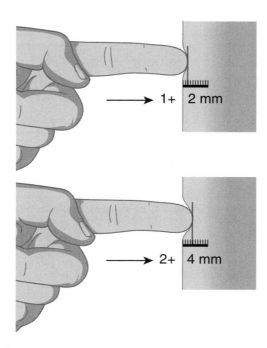

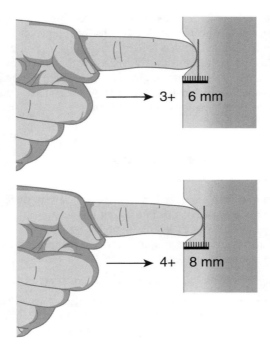

In psychosocial research, questionnaires are often used to quantify personality traits, emotional states, opinions, perceptions, and behaviors. A person's overall anxiety level at any point in time can be measured using a questionnaire with a scale that the responder uses to indicate to what degree each statement is true for them (see **Figure 5-1**). The scores for all the statements are then summed to produce a total score and often separate scores for sub-issues.

- Whether the variable is present or absent
- At what level it is present
- The aspects of the variable that are present
- At what level the aspects are present

Aspects of anxiety could include frequency, degree of perceived threat, physiological sensations, interference with functioning, and duration of the experience. A sub-score for each aspect and a total anxiety score could be calculated. The devices used to measure variables are called tools or instruments. Nursing research instruments commonly include rating scales, questionnaires, physiological measurement, and observational scoring.

In the clinical professions, healthcare providers are interested in the following information about variables of interest:

- Their level (average and range) in various populations.

Example: How much knowledge do middle-age men have regarding the symptoms of heart attack?

- How they change over time.

Circle the number of the phrase that describes your experience of each statement.

My worries interfere with my ability to do my job.

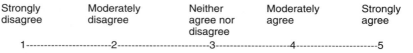

Strongly disagree	Moderately disagree	Neither agree nor disagree	Moderately agree	Strongly agree
1	2	3	4	5

Figure 5-1

Example: How does hope fluctuate across time for women diagnosed with breast cancer?

- How they affect one another.

Example: How does general health affect the exercise level of women in their 60s and 70s?

These interests stem from the nature of clinical practice, which uses information about expected levels, manifestations, and components to diagnose the problems of individual patients and plan preventive, therapeutic, and restorative care for them.

Good Data

In all quantitative research methods, data are considered good when the measurement of variables is consistent and true. Consistent means the measurement method obtains data values very close to each other across repeated testing in the same person, several observers, and various parts of a questionnaire. (Usually, only one of these aspects of consistency is relevant to a particular measurement method.) A consistent measurement method is described in research terms as *reliable*.

A true measurement method captures the essence and attributes of what it is intended to measure. In other words, it zeroes in on the variable of interest and accurately captures it in its totality. When a measurement method accurately captures to a high degree the totality of a variable of interest, researchers say the measure is *valid*. As you will learn, there are several ways of testing a measurement method's **reliability** and **validity**, and the results of these tests are often provided in research reports.

Reliability

Measurement is not as objective as one might think as error and inconsistency can enter into measurement at many points. Consider the clinical situation in which two nurses obtain a blood pressure (BP) on a patient with a stable BP. Assume (1) when the first nurse meets the patient, they are standing at the doorway to the room; (2) the measurements are separated by a 5-minute interval; (3) the second nurse does not know the value the first nurse obtained. Most likely, the two BP values obtained will not be exactly the same, even with digital machines. The difference is probably attributable to variations in their measurement methods more than to changes in the patient's BP. Differences in cuff size, improper application of the cuff, inconsistent patient body position, use of a different arm, arm position, failure to wait before repeating the measurement, and the calibration of the device used can contribute to variation in BP values. In research, differences in readings caused by the difference in measurement technique are considered **measurement error** because the two readings are not identical because of measurement technique as opposed to an actual difference in BP.

To the extent that the BP measurements are obtained using the correct technique each time, they will have less error and will more consistently reflect actual BP. When a measurement method consistently captures the actual value, or is close to it, the measuring method is considered reliable. To increase the reliability of blood pressure measurements in research studies, researchers spell out in great detail the procedure for obtaining and recording a blood pressure measurement to ensure that all persons collecting data do so in the same way.

Specific tests of measurement consistency will be explained in detail as they are used in the exemplar study of this and later chapters.

Validity

A measuring **instrument** may be consistent, but it may fail to capture the essence of the phenomenon of interest. In other words, the measure does not truly measure what it is supposed to measure. Often this is because the variable is difficult to define. For instance, coping with a stressful situation is difficult to define—in contrast to blood pressure, which is much easier to define.

First, consider blood pressure. Conceptually, blood pressure is the pressure generated by the ejection of blood from the left ventricle into the aorta and dispersed throughout the arteries and capillaries. So, blood pressure is a combination of left ventricular ejection force, the arterial system's elastic properties, and the measurement's location relative to the heart's level. The most direct measurement of blood pressure is achieved by placing a small catheter in a peripheral artery and connecting it to a transducer, which senses the pressure, converts it into a waveform, and eventually into a number value. Of course, blood pressure can also be measured indirectly by a blood pressure cuff and sphygmomanometer or nonmercury device. In most situations, indirect BP measurement captures the totality that makes up blood pressure, which is to say that it is a valid measure of what is generally defined as "blood pressure."

In everyday usage, the word *valid* means "true." This is similar to the word's meaning when used to describe a measurement instrument. It is a true (or valid) measure if there is data supporting that it captures in essence and in full the concept it claims to represent. Over the years, a great deal of data supports the high validity of direct blood pressure measurement and the slightly lower validity of indirect BP measurement. The lower validity of indirect BP measurement is because direct BP measurement produces accurate values under a wide range of conditions, including low cardiac output, high peripheral resistance, and patient obesity. However, indirect measurement is either difficult or inaccurate under these conditions. Thus, indirect BP measurement may be valid with some patient populations but have less validity with other populations.

The essence and features of coping are much more difficult to capture than BP. This is partly because coping is a complex, psychological, subjective response of a person over time. It has many features, contextual interactions, and manifestations, whereas blood pressure comprises fewer, readily identified determinants that are very similar in everyone. Also, our understanding of coping is considerably less than our understanding of BP. The result of the complexity, subjective nature, and limited knowledge of coping is that capturing its attributes and diverse manifestations is elusive.

Study participants can be asked to report their level of coping, but the word itself means different things to different persons. Alternatively, the researcher could ask participants to complete a questionnaire to rate various aspects of their daily functioning, emotions, thought processes, sleeping, and eating. A total coping score for each participant could then be produced to reflect various levels of coping. This measurement process sounds comprehensive and straightforward, but the reality is that the questionnaire would have to be developed carefully over time to be sure that it truly captures the many features and manifestations of coping. It would also have to be tested in various populations because it could be valid with some groups of people and not with others. It could be valid with persons with chronic pain but not with persons in a stressful marriage. In short, the measurement of coping is much more complex and much less objective than the measurement of blood pressure.

Measurement of Psychosocial Variables

Measuring psychosocial variables is much trickier than measuring biophysical variables because psychosocial variables do not exist as physical realities. Instead, they exist in individuals' minds, emotions, perceptions, experiences, and behaviors. They also exist conceptually as varying definitions that clinicians, researchers, and theorists assign to them. Thus, psychosocial variables are subjective and intangible—and thus hard to measure.

Often the content of the psychosocial questionnaires and scales used in quantitative research is influenced by earlier qualitative research that identified essential issues. Researchers develop questionnaires, scales, and observation scoring guides to get at the features specified by a particular concept definition. To make questionnaires and scales reliable and valid, researchers revise, develop, and refine them over time, just as the indirect measurement of blood pressure was refined over the years.

It is all too easy for a questionnaire to include features of another psychosocial phenomenon similar to but slightly different from the phenomenon it intends to measure. For example, self-confidence and optimism are concepts that have similarities to—even overlap with—coping. If the questionnaire items are not written carefully, and the balance of items about various features of coping is not correct, some questions might capture self-confidence or optimism instead of coping. Sometimes a physiological measure can be used to indicate a psychological state or behavior. Thus, a physiological, trace indicator of that variable can be measured instead of measuring a psychosocial variable by participant self-report. For instance, salivary cortisol level is used as an indicator of stress and serum glycosylated hemoglobin (HbA1c), which reflects average blood sugar over the past 2 to 3 months (but is heavily weighted to the past 2–4 weeks), is used as an indicator of patient self-management of diabetes. In general, obtaining valid measurements of psychological states is more complex than obtaining valid measurements of physiological states.

Establishing the validity of a psychosocial instrument requires conceptual clarity, testing, comparison with other instruments, and revision. There are many ways of establishing the validity of an instrument. You don't need to know them, but you can be more confident about the validity of an instrument if the researcher reports that checks on the instrument's validity have been performed. Rather than explain how researchers test and report the validity and reliability of instruments, we will explain it in the commentaries about the exemplar studies throughout the text.

> Reliability = Consistency of measurement
> Validity = Accurate capture of underlying concept
> Measurement instrument with high reliability and validity + Sound data
>   collection procedures → Trustworthy data

Extraneous Variables

Before leaving the topic of variables, we want to point out that the researcher decides which variables will be studied when designing a study. Other variables may have influenced the situation but are not of interest in the particular study, and these are referred to as **extraneous variables**—*extraneous* meaning "outside the interest of the study." Even though they are not of interest, if they influence the collected data, they can lead to wrong conclusions. To prevent this, researchers try to anticipate these variables before the study by eliminating or controlling them. *Controlling* means "to isolate, eliminate, or hold steady their influence in the situation."

Let's say that a researcher is interested in studying whether women of different income levels have different receptivity to TV spots about osteoporosis prevention. If the study collects data from a random sample of women ages 15 to 50, age could be an extraneous variable. Thus, even though the data may be analyzed to answer the questions about how income influences receptivity to TV health messages, any differences found could be from a combination of income and age (women with lower incomes might be younger than women with higher incomes). Thus, age is an extraneous variable. It is not of interest in the study, but it may be at work in the situation (e.g., younger women may watch more TV) and could confound the findings—meaning that it confuses or muddies the interpretation of the results.

Recognizing this problem in advance would allow the researcher to conduct the data analysis in a way that considers the effect of age. The researcher could control the age variable by studying only women in a narrower age range, say, 35 to 50 years. The research question would still be about income level and responsiveness to the TV spots, but the influence of age differences would be greatly reduced. However, in the process, the researcher will obtain less information; depending on the research question, this may be okay. Alternatively, statistical methods of analysis could be used to control the effect of age.

One extraneous factor that must always be kept in mind is that in most studies, the participants are aware that they are being studied or that their responses will be examined in detail by the researchers. This may make them think more about issues than they would ordinarily; thus, they may report differently than persons who are not in the study. Another possibility is that the questions asked on a questionnaire influence the person's thinking and change how they answer subsequent questions. Researchers try to minimize the effect of participation in a study, sometimes referred to as the **Hawthorne effect**, by considering the order in which data are collected and/or by giving equal attention to all groups from whom data are collected, so attention doesn't influence participants' responses.

Researchers design studies to gain control over extraneous variables and produce findings regarding the variables that are of genuine interest. However, the world is complex, and it is almost impossible to control all the extraneous variables that are operative in a situation. Therefore, in the report's discussion section, researchers often point out extraneous variables that were not well controlled in their study and may have influenced the findings. Moreover, as clinicians read study reports, they often identify extraneous variables that may have influenced the results—which the researcher was unaware of.

Target Population and Sampling

Ultimately, quantitative research aims to create knowledge about a specified population of people, a population being a large group of persons with characteristics in common (e.g., they all have chronic bone pain after a complex leg fracture). However, data cannot be collected on all persons in the specified population—it is not possible for logistical and cost reasons. Instead, researchers collect data about the variables from a small group of people who are part of the larger population. This smaller group is the **sample**; the group to whom the researchers think their findings are applicable is the target population.

Data are collected from the sample and descriptive statistics are calculated. Even though the statistical results are based on data from one sample, they are the best estimate of what the data might be in the target population. For instance, the mean of the sample is a single-point, best estimate of the target population's mean. In research lingo, we say that the population mean is inferred from the sample mean (**Figure 5-2**).

The flaw of this method of estimating the population mean is that it is based on just one sample. We know that if the researcher obtained other samples from that same population, the mean of each sample would not be exactly the same, but chances are they would not vary widely. Nevertheless, given the fact that data from other samples are not available, the best single-point estimate of the population mean is the mean obtained in the study. However, there is a statistical way of estimating what the means of those other samples from the population might be. It is called a *confidence interval around the sample mean*. It is an interval with specified endpoints between which the means of many other samples from the population are likely to lie. Although it is based on the data from the sample, this interval is highly likely to capture the true population mean. Thus, in Figure 5-1, there is a +/− sign indicating that the inferred population mean is an estimate and the population mean probably is not exactly that value. However, the amount of that +/− value can be estimated from the sample data.

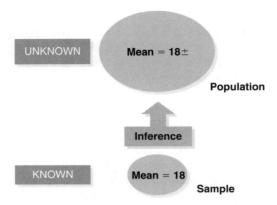

Figure 5-2 Example of Inference

Importantly, for an inference from a sample to a population to be legitimate, the sample must be representative of the population. This means that the sample must be like the population; the sample must match or accurately reflect the population. Any difference could make the inference to the population invalid.

Random Sampling

The very best way to ensure that a sample faithfully represents a population is to randomly select a specified number of persons to be in the sample from the entire population. *Random selection* means that chance alone determines who is selected for the sample. Thus, every person in the population has the same chance of being in the sample. This is possible when a list of the entire membership of a defined population exists, and a method that approximates drawing names out of a hat is used to select who will be in the sample; of course, computer programs, not names in a hat, are most often used to extract a random sample from a list. A sample that is randomly selected from a list of population members is known as a **simple random sample** and usually produces a sample whose profile is very similar to the characteristics of the actual population from which it was drawn. Generally speaking, however, the larger the sample size relative to the population size, the greater the likelihood that the sample will faithfully reflect the population. This method of obtaining a sample and inferring results to the population from which it was drawn is shown graphically in the top diagram of **Figure 5-3**.

Simple Random Sampling

1. Start with a list of all members of the actual population.
2. Randomly draw a sample of predetermined size.
3. Conduct the study with the sample.
4. Make statistical inferences and generalizations to the actual population.

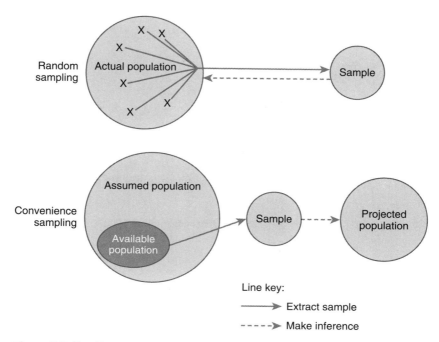

Figure 5-3 Two Types of Population–Sample Relationships

There are several more complicated ways of obtaining a random sample representative of a specified population.

- **Stratified random sampling** is used when the researcher wants to be sure to get data from subgroups of the population that are small and might not be present in sufficient numbers in a simple random sample. The researcher first identifies the relevant strata and their actual percentages in the population. Those percentages determine how many persons are randomly selected from each stratum. Let us say a researcher is interested in studying psychosomatic thinking in diabetics, prediabetics, and nondiabetics and has access to a health center's list of patients. First, the percentages of persons in each of the three strata would be determined. Then, from each stratum, as many persons as needed to maintain the population's strata percentages would be randomly selected to be recruited for the sample. See **Figure 5-4** for an illustration.
- **Cluster sampling** is used when the target population is large and spread out and the researcher needs to concentrate data collection in a few locations. The population is divided into clusters, usually by geographical areas or practice settings, and a specified number of clusters are randomly selected. All persons (or other units of interest) within those clusters are sampled. For instance, if a researcher is interested in collecting data from home care agencies in a state but cannot go all over the state to collect data, five counties in the state could be randomly selected and data collected from all home care agencies in those five counties (**Figure 5-5**).

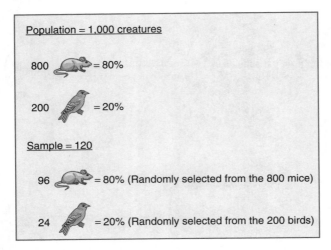

Figure 5-4 Stratified Random Sampling

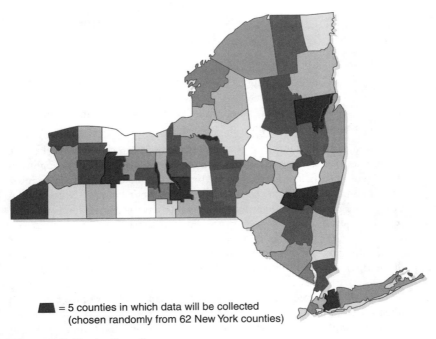

= 5 counties in which data will be collected
(chosen randomly from 62 New York counties)

Figure 5-5 Cluster Sampling

Other methods of random sampling are used but less frequently. So that is all we are going to say about other random sampling methods here. In the future, if you encounter one of them or an unknown (to you) sampling method is in a study report, check out how they are done in a research methods book or via an online search.

Convenience Sampling

In healthcare research, complete lists of population members are quite rare; instead, it is quite common to draw a sample from an available population. Many healthcare studies recruit participants from those available in one or two healthcare agencies. A sample extracted from an available population is a **convenience sample**. To avoid bias, recognized ways of selecting who from the available population will be asked to participate in the study are followed. Convenience sampling starts with an assumed population defined by demographic, disease, functional, symptom, or wellness characteristics. Then, persons are identified who are (1) presumed to be in the assumed population and (2) accessible or available to the researcher; these persons may be accessible in the present or prospectively, that is, going forward. When the study is reported, a detailed profile of the participants, that is, the study sample, is provided; this profile becomes the basis for describing the **projected population** to which statistical conclusions and generalizations can be inferred. Convenience sampling is graphically illustrated in the bottom diagram of Figure 5-2.

Convenience samples reduce the cost and effort of doing a study, but they also introduce the possibility that the study results will not generalize to the target population. There may be something unique about the persons who made up the study sample or the setting in which the study was done that is different from other persons and settings in the assumed population. For this reason, studies with a convenience sample should be replicated in other settings to determine if the results do indeed generalize to others in the assumed population.

Convenience Sampling

1. Specify an assumed population.
2. Identify an available sample of present and/or future persons presumed to be members of the assumed population.
3. Conduct the study with the sample.
4. Develop a detailed profile of the sample's characteristics.
5. Make statistical inferences and generalizations from the study results to a projected population.

Erosion of Representativeness

An important caveat for both random sampling and convenience sampling is that even though the sample selected to be in the study may be representative of the target population, the representativeness of those who contribute data, that is, the *actual* study sample, depends on a high level of consent to participate by those selected to participate and a low level of dropouts once the study is underway. Erosion of representativeness is particularly likely if those who were selected for the sample but declined participation or dropped out have something in common, such as illegal immigration status, transportation difficulties, or language barriers.

Finally, sampling is a broad and complex topic. The preceding explanations just touch on it. Rather than discuss it further here, various methods of obtaining samples and their consequences are discussed in the commentaries of the studies you will read in this and later chapters.

A Target Population Can Be

- The actual population (with a random sample)

                              or

- A projected population (with a convenience sample)

Sample Size

There is no straightforward rule for determining how many participants should be in a **descriptive study**. Earlier, you learned that researchers conducting qualitative studies do not predetermine their sample size; rather, they stop recruiting participants when no new information is forthcoming. In contrast, researchers conducting descriptive studies predetermine their sample sizes by taking into consideration several factors:

- Whether a single group or two groups will be studied
- How the variables will be measured or categorized—that is, whether a mean or a proportion will be calculated
- How much variability is expected in the measurements
- Resources available to conduct the study

Generally, the sample must be large enough that the statistics can precisely estimate the values that groups are likely to exist in the population.

Surveys

A common type of descriptive study is the survey. In surveys, self-reported data are collected by mail, Internet, telephone, or in person. Surveys are widely used because data can be collected from large numbers of people with minimal effort and expense. However, surveys can be misused and subject to different sources of bias, leading to erroneous conclusions (Althubaiti, 2016; Dunsch et al., 2018).

The main problems or sources of bias in surveys are the following:

- Sampling bias: Failure to obtain a sample that is representative of the target population right from the start
- Biased survey questions: Difficulty in constructing questionnaires and interview questions that are clear to everyone who will complete the survey or questions that lead the respondents toward a specific response
- Non-response bias: Low response rates, which make the respondents not representative of the target population (Althubaiti, 2016; Dunsch et al., 2018)

The response rate difficulties of surveys are exemplified in a study of the cardiovascular risk factors and lifestyle habits of preventive cardiovascular nurses (Fair et al., 2009). Emails ($n = 5,163$) were sent to all current and past members of the Preventive Cardiovascular Nurses Association using email addresses from the membership database. A total of 1,358 surveys were completed in the Survey Monkey database, which is a response rate of 26%. The low response rate occurred despite the use of participation enhancement strategies such as early notification, reminders, and incentives. The authors acknowledged the report's low response rate as a study limitation. Unfortunately, the low response rate calls into question the **generalizability** of the findings to the larger population of preventive cardiovascular nurses. This level of response is not uncommon—it can be relatively low for phone, mailed, and emailed online surveys (Amaya & Presser, 2017). Surveys present considerable challenges, but they provide useful information when appropriately conducted. When conducted by the inexperienced, they often produce misleading information.

Results

Percentages

Descriptive studies report results in a variety of ways. Perhaps the most common way is as percentages. For example, a study that measured the impact of fluoroscopy use during radiofrequency ablation with esophageal cooling using a dedicated cooling device in a low-fluoroscopy practice reported that there was a reduction of 35% per case in fluoroscopy time compared with patients who received luminal esophageal temperature monitoring (Zagrodzky et al., 2021).

Center and Spread of the Scores

The mean or median may be reported to convey the typical or representative score. Remember, the mean is the numerical average of the scores and best describes the group average when the scores are evenly distributed around the mean. Means are reported when most of the scores are near the mean, with gradual decreases in the frequency of scores on both sides farther from the mean. The median is the variable value of the middle case and is more typical when the distribution of scores is skewed (i.e., a few scores strung out on *one side* toward the end of the score continuum away from the majority).

For example, in a study that investigated several forms of delay from the onset of symptoms until surgical treatment of spinal metastases for patients with and without a known preexisting known malignancy reported the median patient delay was 19 days, diagnostic delay 21.5 days, referral delay 7 days, and treatment delay 8 days. The median for referral and treatment delay combined was 18.5 days. Comparing patients with and without a known malignancy, the median patient delay was 14 versus 25 days. The authors reported the medians instead of the means for the non-normally distributed data because the distribution was skewed or had outliers rendering unusually low or high values that would render an unrepresentative mean of the data (van Tol et al., 2021).

To convey the variability or spread in the data, researchers often report the range of scores (actual low score and high score) or the interquartile range, which indicates the spread of the middle 50% of scores (see **Figure 5-6**). Data with narrow ranges or interquartile ranges are less dispersed than those with wide ranges. Sometimes data dispersion is of as much interest as is the average of the scores.

Wrap-Up

Percentages, means, medians, and ranges are widely used in reporting the results of descriptive studies. This, plus the natural conditions under which data is collected,

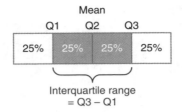

Figure 5-6 Interquartile Range (IQR)

make descriptive studies generally easy to read and understand. Thus, a descriptive study is the first quantitative design to be considered.

Beyond the Study Data

Most often, the researcher conducting quantitative descriptive research aims to present a portrayal of the studied variables as they occurred in the setting and sample in which the study was conducted. Other researchers, however, want to know if their study results would be likely to occur in other similar settings and populations, that is, the larger group of which the sample is only a part. To do this, they use inferential statistics—confidence intervals, chi-square test, *t*-test, ANOVA, and others. However, these tests are not widely used in descriptive studies in nursing so they will not be discussed in this chapter. Inferential statistics will be explained at length in the chapters on correlational research (Chapter 6), experimental research (Chapter 7), and cohort research (Chapter 8).

Exemplar

Reading Tips

This research article is a description of continuous glucose monitoring, the mean amplitude of glycemic excursions in septic patients, and oxidative stress in the intensive care unit. To fully understand the purpose and implications of this study, you should have a basic understanding of the pathophysiology involved in hyperglycemia in critically ill septic patients and the physiologic actions of an insulin infusion. We emphasize that this Profile & Commentary will only make sense if you have read the exemplar article in full and have your completed analysis and application table in front of you.

Exemplar

Quantitative Observational Exemplar

Furushima, N., Egi, M., Obata, N., Sato, H., & Mizobuchi, S. (2021). Mean amplitude of glycemic excursions in septic patients and its association with outcomes: A prospective observational study using continuous glucose monitoring. *Journal of Critical Care, 63*, 218–222. https://doi.org/10.1016/j.jcrc.2020.08.021

Quantitative Observational Analysis and Application Table

		Page
Study Purpose (Why)		
Methods (How)		
Design		
Sample		
Measurement and Quality of Data	Interrater Reliability	
Data Analysis		
Ethics Review		
Results (What)		
Sample		
Findings		
Discussion		

Quantitative Observational Profile and Commentary on the Exemplar Article

Furushima, N., Egi, M., Obata, N., Sato, H., & Mizobuchi, S. (2021). Mean amplitude of glycemic excursions in septic patients and its association with outcomes: A prospective observational study using continuous glucose monitoring. *Journal of Critical Care, 63,* 218–222. https://doi.org/10.1016/j.jcrc.2020.08.021

		Page
Study Purpose (Why)	This study was conducted to apply continuous glucose monitoring (CGM), determine the mean amplitude of glycemic excursions (MAGE) in septic patients, and assess the associations of MAGE with outcomes and oxidative stress.	Abstract p. 218
	The authors then recognize the knowledge gap of there has been no studies investigating associations of oxidative stress in septic patients and glucose variability. They then hypothesized oxidative stress in septic patients is associated with the MAGE.	p. 219
	The takeaway is that hyperglycemia and glucose variability are common in critically ill patients, and insulin infusion is used to avoid hyperglycemia. Literature reports that glucose variability is associated with worse outcomes, and glycemic variability may be an important factor in these critically ill patients. Other studies had limitations in completing glucose measurements (intermittent values). Therefore, the authors propose MAGE and CGM for a more detailed glucose variability.	p. 218

pp. 218–219 |
| | The authors then define oxidative stress. "Oxidative stress is broadly defined as an imbalance of free radicals and other reactive oxygen species or reactive nitrogen species and antioxidant defense systems." Furthermore, they point out that elevated levels of urinary 8-isoPGF2a have been reported in type 2 DM, cardiovascular, degenerative, metabolic, and inflammatory diseases. Lastly, the authors note that no study investigated this association. | |

		Page
Methods (How)		
Design	The study was an observational prospective design at one center. Prospective observational studies are cohort studies that can be prospective or retrospective. A prospective study is carried out from the present time into the future. A positive of prospective studies is that they are designed with specific data collection methods, which gives the advantage of being tailored to collect specific exposure data and may be more complete. The downside of a prospective study is that it may be a long follow-up period while waiting for events or diseases to occur. Thus, this study design is inefficient for investigating diseases with long latency periods and is vulnerable to a high loss to follow-up rate.	p. 219
Sample	This study included 40 ICU patients, which is indicated under "Results." The authors provide inclusion and exclusion criteria in the "patient population and blood glucose control." Inclusion criteria were limited to 1) adult patients, 2) sepsis diagnosis at the time of ICU admission, and 3) expected ICU stay >48 hours. Sepsis was defined according to the sepsis-3 definition. Pregnant patients or patients considered dying were excluded.	p. 219
Measurement and Quality of Data	Evaluation of the quality of observational data is often ignored because it seems straightforward. However, this is not the case for most observational studies. In this study, the authors do not straightforwardly mention the terms "reliability" and "validity" of their measurement tools and procedures because this is a physiological study that uses devices for measurement. However, the steps they took to ensure their data's quality are detailed. First, reliability—these researchers made considerable effort to ensure that they accurately and consistently captured the realities they were observing. In particular, they: ■ Defined the activities of interest in observable terms (blood glucose levels and control, patient information, CGM, MAGE calculation, urinary prostaglandin F2α as a surrogate of oxidative stress)	p. 219

(continues)

		Page

- Based on the continuous insulin infusion according to nurse-driven glucose protocol
- Tested accuracy of the glucose device (Bland-Altman plots)

Second, the validity of measurement instruments is a bit more challenging to assess. First, it is crucial to recognize that the ideal intervals came from existing scientific literature to the extent possible; the authors discussed and provided supporting studies in the materials, methods, and limitations section. So, the validity of these measurement instruments rests in prior scientific work that served as the basis for the ideal time frames. If a new tool was designed for this study, the researchers would have to determine the validity of their observation tool. They would do this by asking experts to look at the tool and determine whether the data to be recorded accurately and comprehensively captures the underlying concepts. Then changes would be made, and a final observation test of the tool would be conducted.

Interrater Reliability

A common way of assessing the reliability of observations is to use interrater reliability. Interrater reliability would be paramount in a study when two or more observers are using a data recording or a scoring instrument. In this study, data was recorded using medical devices, and thus interrater reliability does not apply. However, when a scoring instrument is being used, the observers must be in sync; that is, they record or score the same activity in the same way. If they do not, the data will not be good because it is inconsistent, i.e., it is dependent on who did the recording.

		Page
Data Analysis	The data was analyzed using descriptive statistics: means, medians, ranges, proportions/percentages, correlations, Shapiro-Wilk normality tests, Mann Whitney U test or the chi-square test, and multivariate. Since this study included more than nursing interventions, the researchers ran inferential analyses on their data to check for normality, differences, correlations, accuracy, and adjust for confounders.	p. 219
Ethics Review	The study was reviewed and approved by the institutional review board (IRB) of the involved healthcare organization. An IRB is a group of people appointed by a university, hospital, or other healthcare organization who are responsible for ensuring that human subjects' rights are protected when a study is conducted under their auspices. Federal law requires that IRBs be nationally registered.	Department of Health and Human Services (DHHS), 2022
	A researcher must receive IRB approval before beginning a study and provide reports to the IRB about the ongoing status of the research. In reviewing proposals, IRBs consider the following information:	
	■ How participants will be protected from discomfort and harm and treated with dignity.	
	■ How informed consent (knowledgeable choice to participate or not) will be ensured.	
	■ Whether pressure or coercion to participate in the study is entirely absent.	
	■ How participants in the study will be informed about the purpose of the study, the basis of subject selection, the experimental treatments, assignment to treatment groups, and risks associated with each treatment.	
	■ How privacy, confidentiality, and anonymity will be ensured.	
	Typically the IRB requires an informed consent document to be signed and dated by the participant or the participant's legal guardian. The informed consent document must include a statement giving the researcher access to the participant's	

(continues)

		Page
	protected health information if needed to conduct the study. In some cases, a waiver of signed informed consent may be granted to the researcher due to the low risk for discomfort or harm to the research subjects.	
	By their very nature, some studies involve minimal risk of violating human rights, whereas others are very sensitive. Studies involving infants, children, fetuses, prisoners, reproductive issues, imposed pain or distress, and risks are considered sensitive, and thus the study procedures must be spelled out in great detail (Department of Health and Human Services [DHHS], 2022). Only individuals 18 years or older and legally competent can give their informed consent. Parents or guardians must permit minors to participate. The capacity of persons with cognitive, developmental, and mental health limitations to consent is considered carefully by IRBs.	
	Recognizing the great diversity of studies, an IRB chairperson or committee designates a study as (1) exempt from review, (2) eligible for expedited review, or (3) requiring complete review (DHHS, 2022). The criteria for exempt-from-review status are spelled out in a U.S. Department of Health and Human Services policy. If the risk is minimal, an expedited review can be carried out by the IRB chairperson or by one or more experienced reviewers. A study that has greater than minimal risk must receive a full review by the entire IRB.	
	From this exemplar article, we do not know if this study underwent expedited review or full review; we know that it was approved, and written informed consent was obtained from the patient or a responsible surrogate. Based on IRB approval, we can assume that the patients were assigned subject codes, and their names were not used during data collection and analysis. Also, it is assumed that the principal investigator was the only person with access to the code sheet and ensured its destruction following data collection.	p. 219

		Page
Results (What)		
Sample	The sample comprised 40 ICU patients with 11 non-survivors 90 days after ICU admission. The authors provide a study flow chart in Figure 1. Patient characteristics (age, sex, APACHE ii, septic shock, surgical admission, source of infection, presence of DM) and outcomes (90-day ICU survival days, Urinary 8-isoPGF2a) are provided in Table 1.	pp. 219–220
Findings	Table 2 reports the comparison of blood glucose indices in survivors and non-survivors. Table 2 provides each blood glucose indices' median value, range, percentages, and p-value. Note, in table 2, the p-value for MAGE is 0.02. The authors report in the text that the median value of MAGE was 46.0 mg/dL with the median value of MAGE in non-survivors was 68.8 mg/dL. This was significantly higher than in the survivors ($p = 0.02$).This tells us that higher MAGE is associated with a higher ICU mortality rate. The authors confirmed this significance by checking for normality and using a t-test. No other results in table 2 were statistically significant. However, the authors noted in the text that the non-survivors had higher means when compared to the non-survivors. The authors further note in the "discussion" and "limitations" that because of the small sample size, statistical significance was not reached. They then provide further explanation in the "discussion." It is important to note that even when statistical significance is not obtained, the results can still be clinically important. Researchers should "listen" to the data and not "judge" the findings on statistical significance but also in terms of benefits and harms. Here, the authors have noted that this result has clinical implications which include: using the CGM system the glycemic variability of acute glycemic control could possibly be reached.	pp. 220–221

(continues)

		Page
	Figure 2 reports the relationship between MAGE and urinary 8-isoPGF2α. Figure 2 displays the regression line as a solid line, and dotted lines are 95% confidence intervals. The authors report, non-survivors median urinary 8-isoPGF2α level was not significantly different from the survivors creatinine median value ($p = 0.14$). They report significant MAGE and number of 90-day ICU-free survival days ($p < 0.01$). This tells us that a higher MAGE was associated with fewer ICU-free survival days.	
Discussion	In the discussion section, the researchers compare their results to those of other studies and discuss how the findings of their study are "novel and relevant." They point out that MAGE with outcomes and oxidative stress has not been studied previously, making their study the first to study glycemic variability in patients with sepsis and related outcomes.	pp. 220–221
	The authors mention that prior studies have found that glycemic variability was associated with worse outcomes. Then the authors go on to mention how this study differed in how their study suggests worse outcomes was associated with MAGE and other indices.	
	The authors further explain how MAGE indices versus SD can more accurately reflect glycemic variations.	
	The authors provide clinical implications of their findings: Using a CGM system for evaluation the glycemic variability of acute glycemic control may be reached. Then they offer implications for future research: Future studies should consider using an accurate CGM system to control and evaluate blood glucose levels for evaluating glycemic variability reduction.	
	Lastly, the authors address oxidative stress. They point out that in this study, the MAGE with increased oxidative stress in septic patients association was weak. The authors then connect their results with prior studies, concluding that their results line up with prior study findings.	

		Page
	Limitations are discussed in depth. The authors point out that because of the observational study design, the findings have no causality link. The observational study design should always be listed as a limitation because the design itself makes them more prone to bias and confounding, which cannot be used to demonstrate causality. The authors mention that the small, single center decreases generalizability but that their study should still be considered a preliminary hypothesis-generating study.	

References

Althubaiti, A. (2016). Information bias in health research: Definition, pitfalls, and adjustment methods. *Journal of Multidisciplinary Healthcare, 9*(1), 211–217. https://doi.org/10.2147/JMDH.S104807

Amaya, A., & Presser, S. (2017). Nonresponse bias for univariate and multivariate estimates of social activities and roles. *Public Opinion Quarterly, 81*(1), 1–36. https://doi.org/10.1093/poq/nfw037

Dunsch, F., Evans, D. K., Macis, M., & Wang, Q. (2018). Bias in patient satisfaction surveys: a threat to measuring healthcare quality. *BMJ Global Health, 3*(2), Article e000694. https://doi.org/10.1136/bmjgh-2017-000694

Fair, J., Gulanick, M., & Braun, L. T. (2009). Cardiovascular risk factors and lifestyle habits among preventive cardiovascular nurses. *The Journal of Cardiovascular Nursing, 24*(4), 277–286. https://doi.org/10.1097/JCN.0b013e3181a24375

LaHue, S. C., & Douglas, V. C. (2022). Approach to altered mental status and inpatient delirium. *Neurologic Clinics, 40*(1), 45–57. https://doi.org/10.1016/j.ncl.2021.08.004

Pazar, B., Yava, A., & Başal, Ş. (2015). Health-related quality of life in persons living with a urostomy. *Journal of Wound, Ostomy, and Continence Nursing, 42*(3), 264–270. https://doi.org/10.1097/WON.0000000000000110

van Tol, F. R., Versteeg, A. L., Verkooijen, H. M., Öner, F. C., & Verlaan, J.-J. (2021). Time to surgical treatment for metastatic spinal disease: Identification of delay intervals. *Global Spine Journal,* 2192568221994787. https://doi.org/10.1177/2192568221994787

Zagrodzky, J., Bailey, S., Shah, S., & Kulstad, E. (2021). Impact of active esophageal cooling on fluoroscopy usage during left atrial ablation. *The Journal of Innovations in Cardiac Rhythm Management (Print), 12*(11), 4749–4755. https://doi.org/10.19102/icrm.2021.121101

CHAPTER 6

Correlational Research

Another form of quantitative research goes beyond reporting basic facts about a variable of interest to explore how variables are related to one another. Questions include: Is spousal or partner support associated with diabetics' blood sugar levels? Are levels of hearing loss and levels of osteoporosis related? Do lung capacity levels predict exercise capacity? These questions ask, "Are variable X and variable Y related?" or "Do their levels move in sync to some extent?" These questions go beyond a description of each variable separately to examine the relationship between them. They are the kinds of questions that can be answered by **correlational research**.

Defining *Relationship*

Just what does the word *relationship* mean in the research context? In simplest terms, a relationship describes an association between two sets of scores. Let's say, from each person in a sample of 30–40-year-olds; the researchers collected two pieces of data: their heart rate after 5 minutes on a treadmill and their body mass index (BMI). If there is a strong trend for those with low 5-minute heart rates to have low BMIs and those with high 5-minute heart rates to have high BMIs, the two variables would be considered to be associated, that is, correlated, in the sample. Notably, the association says nothing about the dynamics that link them—just that they are connected in some way. Establishing the dynamics would require a persuasive theory and other research.

A relationship has two dimensions—direction and strength. The direction of change can be in the same direction or opposite directions. In a positive relationship, as one variable's values increase, the other's values increase as in the example just given. In a negative relationship, as one variable's values increase, the other's values decrease; for example, in a test situation, scores on the test decrease as anxiety levels rise.

A relationship can also be characterized as strong, moderate, or weak, indicating the strength of the relationship between the two variables. A positive relationship is strong when:

1. Persons who score high on variable A also score high on variable B *and*
2. Persons who score low on variable A also score low on variable B *and*
3. Those who score intermediate on variable A also score intermediate on variable B.

Note that each of these statements could also be stated in the inverse; for example, persons who score high on *B* also score high on *A*. By contrast, a weak relationship exists when:

1. Just a few persons who score high on *A* also score high on *B,* but quite a few others score medium or low on *B and*
2. Just a few persons who score low on *A* also score low on *B,* but quite a few others score medium or high on *B and*
3. Those who score intermediate on *A* have assorted scores on *B.*

In other words, the relationship is weak when there is very little connection between persons' scores on *A* and scores on *B.*

The opposite of *relationship* is **independence**, meaning there is no association between scores on the two variables. There is no pattern in the scores of one variable with the scores on the other variable; both are scattered across the range of possible scores. A pattern or lack thereof is best seen by plotting the data points on a graph with values of *A* on one axis and values of *B* on the other axis—there will either be a degree of trend or a wide scatter, as you will see in the next section.

Measuring a Relationship

Statistical Perspectives on Relationship

The direction and strength of a relationship between two variables are quantified using several statistical tests. The actual statistic depends on the scale used to quantify the variables. When both variables were measured on an interval level scale, the **Pearson r coefficient** is used; it is the most widely used **correlation** statistic (Gray & Grove, 2021). An interval level scale is a measurement scale with a range of numerical values having equal distance between them, such as degrees on a thermometer or pounds on a weight scale. If either or both variables are measured using an ordered set of categories, for example, *freshman, sophomore, junior, senior,* the Pearson *r* coefficient is not used; rather, another correlation coefficient would be used. There are several, but they all are interpreted similarly to the interpretation of the Pearson *r* coefficient.

The value of the Pearson *r* statistic varies from −1 to +1, which means that it can be: −1, a negative decimal, 0, a positive decimal, or +1. The sign indicates whether the two variables have a positive or negative relationship; if positive, they move in the same direction; if negative, they move in opposite directions. The closer the value is to −1 or +1, the stronger the relationship between the two variables. Zero means the two variables are entirely independent of one another, and a value close to 0 (e.g., +0.2) indicates a very weak relationship.

Interpretation of *r*							
r-value	−1	−0.8	−0.5	0	+0.6	+0.8	+1
relationship	perfect negative	strong neg	moderate neg	none	moderate positive	strong pos	perfect pos

Graph Perspectives on a Relationship

To illustrate relationship in the concrete, a hypothetical study (**BOX 6-1**) and five possible data sets for the study are presented in the following figures (**Figures 6-1** through **6-5**). Each data set is accompanied by a scatter plot for the data, the Pearson *r* coefficient for the data, and explanations about what these two analytical tools tell us. The samples in the data sets were limited to five scores to make it easier to see the relationship between the two variables, although an actual study would not have as few as five cases. If you are not up to speed regarding scatter plots, also called scatter diagrams, you should go back and read about them in your statistics reference text. You will not see many scatter plots in journal reports because they take up too much room, but they help identify trends in data and many researchers will mention them in the text.

Box 6-1 **Hypothetical Correlational Study**

Study Purpose:
To examine the relationship between hope and adaptation in persons who have had multiple sclerosis for at least 3 years.

Measurement
On two short questionnaires, total hope scores can range from 0 to 5. A score of 0 = no hope and 5 = an abundance of hope; and total adaptation scores can range from 0 to 10, with 0 = not able to function independently in daily life and 10 = functioning without problems. Note that both variables are scored on continuous scales; this is a key requirement for using the Pearson *r* correlation coefficient to portray the relationship between the two variables. If one variable is continuous (e.g., adaptation) but the other is categorical (e.g., gender), the Pearson *r* statistic could not be used.

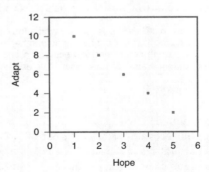

Sample:
Five people

Results
Several possible scores are presented in Figures 6-1 through 6-6. To make the relationship between the variables stand out, the hope scores are the same from data set to data set, but the adaptation scores are different.

Dataset 1	Person	Hope score	Adaptation score
	1	1	2
	2	2	4
	3	3	6
	4	4	8
	5	5	10

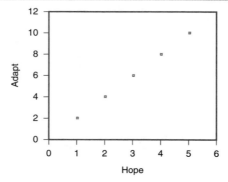

Note that for each increase of 1 point in hope scores, there is a 2-point increase in the adaptation scores. If you know a person's hope score, you can accurately predict that person's adaptation score; similarly if you know the person's adaptation score, you can accurately predict his or her hope score. When two variables change in lockstep with one another, we say that they have a perfect positive correlation. There is nothing magical about the 1-point-hope score to 2-point-adaptation score relationship. It could just as easily be that a 1-point change in hope is related to a 4-point change in adaptation; it depends on the scales used to measure the two variables.

Note that scatter plots provide the same information as the data set table. Each point on the scatter plot represents one score. For example, the person who scored 10 on hope scored 20 on adaptation and has a point on the scatter plot as does the person who scored 40 on hope and 80 on adaptation. Because the relationship between the two variables is in lockstep, a line drawn between all the data points is a straight line.

The Pearson r statistic for this data set is $r = +1$, which indicates a perfect positive relationship. The two variables move in lockstep with one another with high scores on one being paired with high scores on the other and low scores on one being paired with low scores on the other. The Pearson r statistic has possible values between +1 and −1.

Figure 6-1 Hypothetical Data Set 1

Perfect correlations are, of course, a rare happening in the real world where variation and multiple influences are characteristic of reality, especially in the social, psychological, and behavioral realms. Instead, weak, moderate, and moderately strong correlations occur more often. These relationships are illustrated in the three hypothetical data sets (Figures 6-3, 6-4, and 6-5).

In summary, a correlation coefficient indicates the direction (positive or negative) and strength (perfect, strong, moderate, weak, or none) of a relationship.

Caveat

Again, a strong relationship between two variables says nothing about the underlying dynamic that produces the relationship. A very high correlation (near −1 or +1) does not mean a cause-and-effect relationship between the variables. The high

Dataset 2	Person	Hope score	Adaptation score
	1	1	10
	2	2	8
	3	3	6
	4	4	4
	5	5	2

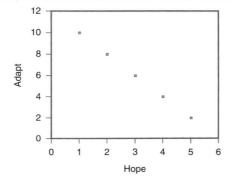

Note that for each increase of 1-point in hope score there is a 2-point decrease in adaptation score. Just as in data set 1, if you know a person's hope score, you can accurately predict that person's adaptation score; similarly if you know the person's adaptation score, you can accurately predict his or her hope score. However, instead of moving in the same direction as they did in data set 1, they move in the opposite direction. The variables in this data set have a perfect negative relationship: As one variable goes up, the other goes down in lockstep a specific amount. Again, a line drawn between all the data points is a straight line. The Pearson r-value for this data set is $r = -1$, indicating a perfect negative relationship.

Figure 6-2 Hypothetical Data Set 2

correlation only conveys a pattern in the relationship between the two variables. The relationship between the two variables could be much more complex than straightforward cause and effect.

For instance, look at Figure 6-3 again. At first glance, the scatter plot and the Pearson r of 0.93 seem to suggest that level of hope determines the level of adaptation. However, identical data could be found if the reverse were true; successful adaptation generates hope. Another possibility is that the relationship between the two variables is not direct. There could be another lurking variable in the background that strongly affects both hope and adaptation and causes them to move in concert with one another; that lurking variable could be something like prognosis or response to treatment. In any of these three dynamics, the data and the Pearson r-value could be the same as in Figure 6-3. The point is this: Correlation sheds no light on the dynamics underlying the relationship even when one precedes the other in time. Correlation analysis only detects a relationship. The dynamics of that relationship need to be ferreted out by further research using other research designs or justified by other knowledge about the two phenomena.

Dataset 3	Person	Hope score	Adaptation score
	1	1	2
	2	2	3
	3	3	6
	4	4	9
	5	5	8

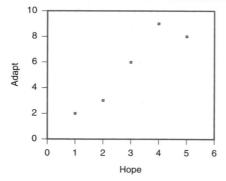

Note that an increase in hope is roughly related to an increase in adaptation. The two variables are strongly but not perfectly correlated. If you know a person's score on one variable, you can make a pretty good estimate of the person's score on the other variable.

A trend in the data is quite obvious, but all the data points are not in a straight line. If a straight line were drawn through the middle of the data, three data points would be on or very close to that line and two would be a bit farther away. The line is called the *trend line* and represents the middle of the data. Take a straight edge and add a trend line to this graph.

The Pearson *r* coefficient for this data set is +0.93, which is a strong, positive correlation.

Figure 6-3 Hypothetical Data Set 3

When the relationship between age and vitamin D was assessed, the Pearson *r* was 0.071. The authors interpreted this result that vitamin D levels did not have a significant correlation with maternal age (Ahi et al., 2022).

Outliers

When looking at scatter plots, the researcher looks for **outliers**, which are cases with very atypical score pairings. An outlier's data point will lie very far from the trend line. Importantly, a single outlier can considerably lower the Pearson *r* with small sample sizes. Consider the scatter plot in **Figure 6-6**. Most of the scores lie close to the positive correlation trend line, except for the person who scored 40 on hope and 10 on adaptation. This person's data is an outlier because it is very different from the other scores. The Pearson *r* for this data set is 0.50, which is a medium correlation. However, reanalysis produces a Pearson r of 0.98 for the other four scores when this outlier is removed. The Pearson *r* calculated with the outlier left in is greatly influenced because the sample size is so small; still, studies with larger sample sizes can be moderately influenced by a single outlier.

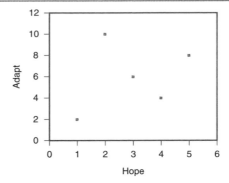

Dataset 4	Person	Hope score	Adaptation score
	1	1	2
	2	2	10
	3	3	6
	4	4	4
	5	5	8

There is a bit of a linear trend in the relationship between hope and adaptation; as hope scores go up, there is a bit of a trend for the adaptation score to go up, but the relationship is weak. Any effort to base one score on the other score would have a low likelihood of being accurate.

A trend line drawn through the middle of the data would show that three data points are on or close to the trend line, but two are quite far from it. Thus, there is a trend, but a weak one. The Pearson r coefficient for this data set is +0.30, indicating a moderately weak positive correlation.

Figure 6-4 Hypothetical Data Set 4

An outlier can either understate or exaggerate the strength of the relationship between the two variables, depending on the values that make up the outlier. Removing an outlier or several in a data set can uncover a trend that would be less clear if the outliers were left in. When researchers remove data for analysis, they should do so with sound rationale and acknowledge that they did so. Removing data could be a form of bias, particularly when the study has a small sample size. Sometimes, a researcher will examine outlier cases in great depth because doing so can yield valuable insights that set the agenda for future research.

Practical Perspectives on *r*-Value

Even though an r of 1.00 indicates a perfect positive relationship between hope and adaptation in which the variables move in lockstep with one another, an r-value of 0.70 does *not* mean that 70% of the values of hope move in lockstep with adaptation; rather, the r-value indicates the relative strength of the relationship on a scale from −1 to +1. Huck (2011) points out that r exaggerates how strong the relationship is between two variables. A more realistic and practical perspective is gained by squaring the value of r to produce r^2, called the **coefficient of determination**. The r^2 value indicates the percentage of variation in hope related to adaptation and the percentage of variation in adaptation related to hope (see **Figure 6-7**). When an r of 0.70 is squared, yielding an r^2 of 0.49, this tells us that about half the variation

Dataset 5	Person	Hope score	Adaptation score
	1	1	7
	2	2	3
	3	3	10
	4	4	5
	5	5	6

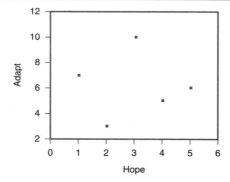

In this data set, there is no relationship between the hope score and the adaptation score; the two scores are independent of one another. Knowing one score will not enable you to predict the other one. All data points are quite far from a trend line drawn through the data. The Pearson r coefficient for this data set is 0, indicating no relationship between the two variables.

Figure 6-5 Hypothetical Data Set 5

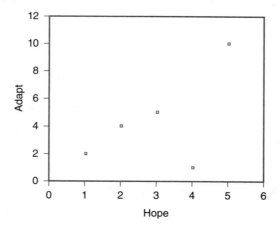

The Pearson r for this data set is 0.50, indicating a modest association. The outlier has lowered an otherwise high Pearson r-value. It pulls the r statistic down a lot because the data set is so small.

Figure 6-6 Example of Outlier

in hope is related to adaptation, and half of the variation in adaptation is related to hope. The other 51% of both variables is attributable to other, often unknown, influences. In short, r^2 provides a more practical sense of the strength of the relationship between the two variables than r itself.

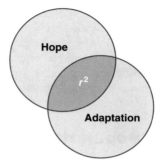

r^2 indicates the amount of variability in each variable that is explained by the other variable. The rest is explained by other, often unknown, influences.

Figure 6-7 r^2

Correlational Design

Bivariate Analysis

The most straightforward correlational design is when the relationship between two or more variables is studied in a sample of people. The researcher measures the participants on each of the variables of interest using instruments that have been established as reliable and valid with the population under study. No attempt is made to control or manipulate the situation. As with descriptive studies, good data are key to a good study; thus, most researchers report information about the reliability and validity of the instruments they use. The data analysis consists of running correlational tests to determine if and how the variables are related. In basic correlational studies, the analysis measures the strength of the association between various combinations of two variables, called **bivariate correlation**. If there are three variables in the study, *A*, *B*, and *C*, bivariate analysis could be run on the relationship between *A* and *B*, *A* and *C*, and *B* and *C*, thus producing three correlation coefficients.

Some of the variables included in a study come from the hunches of clinicians practicing in the area; others come from theory or related academic work. Often, researchers conduct correlational studies to explore clinical issues that are murky, such as:

- What factors influence young women's positive adaptation to having human papilloma virus (HPV)?
- What factors influence a double amputee's motivation in rehabilitation?

Correlational studies help identify promising ideas for future research, whereas others may demote ideas that did not hold up.

Although correlational studies cannot establish a connection between cause and effect, there are times when results from correlational studies make a strong case for cause and effect. This would be the case when experimental design cannot be used. An example might be studying the possible relationship between maternal gum disease and infant preterm low birth weight. Researchers cannot randomly assign mothers to have gum disease prior to or during pregnancy. Moreover, if a study found a high correlation between gum disease and low birth weight, a third factor may have influenced the development of both conditions such as poor diet, smoking, or alcohol consumption. It would also be prudent to keep in mind that a single determinant does not cause most health conditions and that several determinants often interact with each other to cause a condition. To claim that maternal gum disease causes infant low birth weight would require cohort studies and a credible theory regarding the causative mechanism, but a correlational study could be a starting point for examining the issue. Cohort studies are examined in Chapter 8.

Generalizing to a Population

Researchers can go beyond statistically estimating the relationship among the variables in the sample studied to educated guesses about whether the relationships will also be found in a population with a similar profile. The statistical analysis that analyzes each bivariate relationship produces an r statistic and a data-based p-value. If this **p-value** is less than the preset, critical p-value (i.e., it is significant), it indicates that the population's correlation is not zero. Importantly, it does *not* indicate that the correlation between the two variables in the population is of the same strength as was found in the sample. Nor does it indicate that the relationship is particularly strong. It signals that the two variables are related to some degree (positively or negatively depending on the sign of r) in the population. If the data-based p-value produced by the analysis is greater than the critical **p-level** (i.e., not significant), the correlation between the two variables in the population likely is zero (see **Figure 6-8**).

Further explanation of p-value interpretation is provided in the *Profile & Commentary* on the exemplar article of this chapter. Seeing it in context may make it clearer to you.

More Complex Designs

So far, this chapter has focused on the simplest type of correlational study, but there are more powerful ones. Complex correlational designs collect data on a few variables to determine the combination of variables that best *predict* the level of an outcome variable of interest. One such design uses **multiple regression analysis** to determine which *set* of predictor variables best predicts the level of an outcome variable. Using a statistical program, predictor variable values are entered into the analysis one at a time until the combination of variables that best predicts levels of the outcome variable is found. The amount of variability among the outcome

Data-based p-value	< .001	.01	.025	**.05**	.08	.15	.42 >
Finding	Significant correlation				Nonsignificant correlation		
Conclusion	A correlation of zero may be found in the population.				A correlation of greater or less than zero would likely be found in the population.		

*Using a .05 level of significance decision point

Figure 6-8 Interpretation of p-Values Associated with Pearson r

variable scores explained by the best set of predictor variables is quantified as the R^2 statistic.

For example, a study examined the association between depression, anxiety, and self-esteem in older people living in nursing homes. The Patient Health Questionnaire (PHQ-9) was used to evaluate depression levels, the Generalized Anxiety Disorder Scale (GAD-7) was used to measure anxiety levels, and self-esteem was tested by the Rosenberg Self-Esteem Scale (RSES). Each instrument is a scale that produced a depression, anxiety, and self-esteem level score. A significant positive correlation was found between anxiety and depression ($R = 0.75$; $p < 0.001$). A negative moderate correlation was found between self-esteem and anxiety ($R = -0.50$; $p < 0.001$) and between self-esteem and depression ($R = -0.63$; $p < 0.001$). This means the higher the depression level was in older people, the lower their self-esteem and the higher their anxiety (Šare et al., 2021).

Outcome Prediction

Other studies use predictor variables to distinguish between the prevalence of categorical outcomes (e.g., quit smoking/did not quit smoking; occurrence/nonoccurrence); a widely used statistical technique for this purpose is **logistic regression**. Whereas multiple regression is used when the outcome variable is continuous, logistic regression is used when the outcome variable is categorical. The results are reported using a measure called **odds ratio**.

An odds ratio (OR) compares the likelihood of two or more independent variables (cause) association between an exposure and an outcome. For example, it could be used to quantify the factors (exposure) that contribute to patient falls (outcome) in the hospital setting. Fall or did not fall is the dependent (outcome) variable of the analyses. Independent variables (cause or exposure) could include narcotics, fall prevention strategy, age, and bedrest. An odds ratio of 1 or near 1 indicates that there is no association between exposure and outcome between groups (case-patients and controls). An odds ratio greater than 1 indicates that the odds of exposure among case-patients are greater than the odds of exposure among controls, meaning the exposure could be a risk factor. An odds ratio less than 1 indicates that the odds of exposure among case-patients are lower than the odds of exposure among controls, meaning the exposure could be a protective factor. Using the example above, when narcotics are prescribed, the odds ratio was 18.24 (OR = 18.24) for a fall. This indicates that the patients prescribed narcotics were 18 times more likely to fall than patients who were not prescribed narcotics.

In a study by Zhang, Si, and Pi (2021) stepwise multiple logistics regression was used to determine the factors associated with the fear of falling in older patients after total knee arthroplasty (TKA). The independent variables were factors that differed significantly between patients reporting or not reporting fear, while the dependent variable was fear of falling (treated as a binary variable). Many variables were analyzed, but only three of them were independent risk factors for fear of falling.

- Female sex TKA patients had an odds ratio of 4.21 (OR = 4.21) for fear of falling, indicating that female patients with TKA were 4.2 times more likely to fear falling than males.
- Having a greater BMI or being an obese TKA patient had an odds ratio of 3.93 (OR = 3.93) for fear of falling, indicating that obese TKA patients were 3.9 times more likely to fear falling than non-obese TKA patients.

- Higher anxiety among TKA patients had an odds ratio of 1.56 (OR = 1.56) for fear of falling, indicating that TKA patients with higher anxiety levels were one and a half times more likely to fear falling than TKA patients with lower levels of anxiety.

Most studies use logistic or multiple regression as the main methods of correlational analysis. Therefore, it is essential that you have a statistics book for reference.

Exemplar

Quantitative Correlational Exemplar Article

Parizad, N., Goli, R., Mirzaee, R., Baghaie, R., & Habibzadeh, H. (2021). Satisfaction with nursing care and its related factors in patients with COVID-19: A descriptive correlational study. *Journal of Education and Health Promotion, 10*, Article 437. https://www.ncbi.nlm.nih.gov/pmc/articles/PMC8719559

WWW

Quantitative Correlational Analysis and Application Table

		Page
Study Purpose (Why)		
Methods (How)		
Design		
Sample		
Measurement and Quality of Data	**Interrater Reliability**	
Data Analysis		

		Page
Ethics Review		
Results (What)		
Sample		
Findings		
Discussion		

Quantitative Correlational Profile and Commentary on the Exemplar Article

Parizad, N., Goli, R., Mirzaee, R., Baghaie, R., & Habibzadeh, H. (2021). Satisfaction with nursing care and its related factors in patients with COVID-19: A descriptive correlational study. *Journal of Education and Health Promotion, 10,* Article 437. https://www.ncbi.nlm.nih.gov/pmc/articles/PMC8719559

		Page
Study Purpose (Why)	This study's aim was to determine what patients with COVID-19 satisfaction and related factors were.	Abstract
	The authors further state research questions "1. What is the patient's satisfaction level of patients with COVID-19 from nursing care? 2. What factors do affect the patient's satisfaction in patients with COVID-19?"	p. 2

(continues)

		Page
Methods (How)		
Design	The authors describe this study as a "descriptive correlational study." The study is correlational because the researchers investigate relationships between variables without the researcher controlling or manipulating them. The study is also descriptive because the research aims to accurately and systematically describe a population, situation, or phenomenon.	p. 2
Sample	The sample comprised 196 patients with COVID-19 in clinical wards of Taleghani Hospital in Urmia. The authors estimated sample size of 196 patients based on a previous study, the patient satisfaction ratio ($P = 0.85$), maximum error level ($d = 5\%$), and confidence level ($1 - \alpha =0.95$). The authors list inclusion criteria 1) must be between 18–60 years of age, 2) willing to participate, 3) orientated and capable of reading and writing, 4) no vision or hearing problems, 5) no mental health history, and 6) $SPO_2 > 90\%$. The authors used convenient purposive sampling, meaning the sample was conveniently accessible to the researchers and purposive because the sample was chosen based on their characteristics that fit the purpose of the study.	pp. 2–3
Measurement and Quality of Data	The report provides quite a bit of information about the Patient Satisfaction Instrument (PSI) to assure the readers of the reliability and validity. The authors recognize that the instrument used was developed by Hinshaw and Atwood (1982). The instrument consisted of 25 items, with a 5-point Likert scale ranging from totally agree to totally disagree. The minimum score was 25 and maximum score was 125. Dissatisfaction was a score <78 and moderate satisfaction was a score between 78 and 104 and complete satisfaction was a score > 104. The instrument was divided into 3 subscales: 1) knowledge, carefulness, and technical skills; 2) nurse-patient relationship; and 3) education.	pp. 2–3

		Page
	Reliability	
	Of note, beyond the original authors, since then, the PSI instrument has been used, and its reliability and validity has been established. The authors do a great job of referencing Akre et al. (2010) for the sensitivity of the PIS being 80% and then reference Jagoda et al. (2019) who used Cronbach's alpha to confirm the instrument's reliability (α =0.88). Cronbach's alpha is a measure of internal consistency, that is, how closely related a set of items are as a group. It is considered to be a measure of scale reliability. The closer Cronbach's alpha coefficient is to 1.0, the greater the internal consistency of the items in the scale. So a value above 0.80 is a very good level and would indicate that together the items capture the satisfaction of technical-professional care, trust, and patient education. A Cronbach's alpha at 0.60–0.70 is an acceptable level; however, it introduces concern that some items of the instrument are not focused on the same concept as the others.	
	Validity	
	The content validity determined the validity of this PSI instrument. The authors point out that for this study, the questionnaire was in both, English and Persian language. The questionnaire was dristributed to 10 faculty members at the Urmia University of Medical Sciences, Nursing and Midwifery. The faculty members, opions and comments were collected for analysis.	
	The authors then reference previous studies again that established validity and reliability of the questionnaire had been confirmed by previous studies in Iran (Jannati et al., 2016; Peyrovi et al., 2013). They then mention that "test and re-test method was used to confirm the reliability of the questionnaire and the correlation coefficient was 0.92." Test-retest reliability measures the consistency of the results when you repeat the same test on the same sample at a different point in time.	
	The authors then provide detailed information on how data collection occurred; a questionnaire was filled out based on direct interviews with a nurse being the interviewer who worked directly with the COVID-19 patients on the ward. They also mention the safety measures set in place for data collection.	

(continues)

		Page
Data Analysis	Descriptive and inferential statistics (frequency, percentages, mean, and SD), Kolmogorov–Smirnov, and Pearson correlation were used for the analysis.	p. 3
Ethics Review	The study was approved by the research and ethics committee of Urmia University of Medical Science. The authors provided the approval number: IR. UMSU.REC.1399.136.	p. 3
Results (What)		
Sample	The demographic characteristics of the sample and their correlation with patient satisfaction is reported in Table 1. Note that this sample had more male, employed, high school education level, married, urban, non-smoking, and enough income level.	pp. 3–4
Findings	**Associations** Then comes the correlational part of the results. The Pearson correlation test was used to assess patient satisfaction and related factors in patients with COVID-19. Table 1 presents the correlation results in the right column (p, r). Pearson correlation is represented with a '*'. Now, recall a correlation of −1 shows a perfect negative correlation, while a correlation of 1 shows a perfect positive correlation. A correlation of 0 shows no relationship between the movement of the two variables; this is a	pp. 3–4
	negligible correlation. Glancing at table 1, you can see all r values, except 1 (residential status) are 0, meaning the correlation of these factors is so small that they are insignificant. **Inference from Sample to Population** The authors ran a test of significance with Pearson correlation. Recall that the significant p-values in the context of correlation statistics indicate whether or not the correlation is likely to be zero in a larger population. In Table 1, you can see that one factor, residential status ($p = 0.001$) is significant, meaning $p < 0.05$. Although the authors did not specifically state what value they were accepting as significant, a $p < 0.05$ is most often used. Residential status was found to have a significant inverse relationship with COVID-19 patient satisfaction level ($p = 0.001$). In this case, the inverse correlation means that residential status was correlated with a decrease in satisfaction level.	

		Page
Discussion	In the discussion section, the researchers compare their results to those of other studies. They link their results as being consistent with other studies. They discuss how the residential status differed from previous studies. The authors point out potential extraneous variables, the variables you're not investigating that can potentially affect the outcomes of your research study. They note that that within various countries, patients' satisfaction can be influenced by extraneous factors and attempts to solve them is crucial.	pp. 4–5
	They then link their statement to another study by recognizing that the findings could be rooted in the patients low expectations of the healthcare services.	
	Limitations	
	The authors acknowledged the limitations of their study. They note the extraneous variables as psychosocial, behavioral and environmental. The researchers have no control over the exranous variables, thus have the potential of influencing the patients' satisfaction scores.	
	Generalizability is a limitation because their study was only conducted at a single hospital. Lastly, the authors give direction for future research, expand to more than one hospital, and assess satisfaction with nursing care in outpatients with COVID-19.	

References

Ahi, S., Adelpour, M., Fereydooni, I., & Hatami, N. (2022). Correlation between maternal vitamin d and thyroid function in pregnancy with maternal and neonatal outcomes: A cross-sectional study. *International Journal of Endocrinology, 2022*, Article 6295775. https://doi.org/10.1155/2022/6295775

Akre, M., Finkelstein, M., Erickson, M., Liu, M., Vanderbilt, L., & Billman, G. (2010). Sensitivity of the pediatric early warning score to identify patient deterioration. *Pediatrics (Evanston), 125*(4), e763–e769. https://doi.org/10.1542/peds.2009-0338

Gray, J. R., & Grove, S. K. (2021). Burns and Grove's *The practice of nursing research: Appraisal, synthesis, and generation of evidence* (9th ed.). Elsevier Saunders.

Hinshaw, A., & Atwood, J. R. (1982). A patient satisfaction instrument: Precision by replication. *Nursing Research (New York), 31*(3), 170–175. https://doi.org/10.1097/00006199-198205000-00011

Huck, S. W. (2011). *Reading statistics and research* (6th ed.). Pearson.

Parizad, N., Goli, R., Mirzaee, R., Baghaie, R., & Habibzadeh, H. (2021). Satisfaction with nursing care and its related factors in patients with COVID-19: A descriptive correlational study. *Journal of Education and Health Promotion, 10*, Article 437. https://www.ncbi.nlm.nih.gov/pmc/articles/PMC8719559

Šare, S., Ljubičić, M., Gusar, I., Čanović, S., & Konjevoda, S. (2021). Self-esteem, anxiety, and depression in older people in nursing homes. *Healthcare (Basel), 9*(8), Article 1035. https://doi .org/10.3390/healthcare9081035

Zhang, H., Si, W., & Pi, H. (2021). Incidence and risk factors related to fear of falling during the first mobilisation after total knee arthroplasty among older patients with knee osteoarthritis: A cross-sectional study. *Journal of Clinical Nursing, 30*(17–18), 2665–2672. https://doi .org/10.1111/jocn.15731

CHAPTER 7

Experimental Research

Chapter Map

This is a very long chapter; therefore, it is divided into two main sections. The first section focuses on the methods used to conduct **experimental studies** testing the effectiveness of nursing **interventions**. The second section delves into the ways the results of experimental studies are reported.

In the first section, the methodological characteristics of experimental studies are explained, followed by a break to complete section 1 of the exemplar article analysis and application table. It would be best if you read only the *Introduction* and *Material and Methods* sections of the exemplar study, then read the *Profile & Commentary* about its methods. The second section opens with an explanation of the results of experimental studies. After reading that, you should read the *Results* section of the exemplar study and then the *Profile & Commentary* about its results. In other words, rather than ingest the whole research article at once, you will first consider the *why* and the *how*. Then you will delve into the *what*. When you see the amount of information in this chapter, you will understand why it is divided into two portions.

The explanations in this chapter will be limited to the classic two-group experiment, which is widely used in nursing research. Although in the future, you will undoubtedly read three-group experimental studies, you should be able to understand them using what you know about two-group studies and by referencing your statistics book. This text does not address other experimental designs that are used less often.

The classic experimental study discussed in this chapter is also referred to in healthcare research as a **randomized clinical trial (RCT)**. Having said that, some people view an RCT more narrowly as a definitive, late-stage test of an intervention's effectiveness, often in a large, diverse sample (Gray & Grove, 2021).

Chapter Layout

Section 1

- Methods explained
- Exemplar study: Read Introduction and Material and Methods sections only
- Profile & Commentary: Why and How

Section 2

- Results explained
- Exemplar study: Read Results and Discussion sections
- Profile & Commentary: What

Section 1: Experimental Methods

Determining the effectiveness of nursing interventions and treatments requires carefully designed studies. Assembling a group of willing participants and measuring them on a physiologic condition, psychological state, or knowledge level before and after receiving the intervention of interest is considered a weak design (Curtis et al., 2018). It is weak because if an improvement is found, the researcher cannot claim with certainty that the intervention produced the improvement. Natural recovery, natural fluctuations in condition, or influences in the environment may have caused the observed improvements. Adding a **control group** that is also measured before and after allows these extraneous influences to be considered.

Key Features of Experimental Studies

When researchers want to test the effects of a nursing intervention on patient outcomes, the ideal research design is an experiment. A sample is drawn from a target population, and participants are randomly assigned to one of two groups. One group receives the test intervention and the other receives no intervention. At an appropriate time after the intervention, the researcher measures an outcome variable, or several, in both groups to determine whether one group did better (see **Figure 7-1**). In designing an experimental study, the researcher tries to create conditions in which all influences on the outcome of interest, other than the effects of the different interventions, are the same for both groups. This sameness is necessary to be sure that any difference found in the outcomes of the two groups can be attributed to the fact that they received different interventions, not to some other influence.

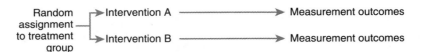

Figure 7-1 Classic Two-Group Experimental Study Sequence

The classic experimental study has six key features:

1. A well-defined target population
2. Adequate sample size
3. **Random assignment** of participants to intervention and **comparison groups**
4. Control of extraneous influences and bias
5. Low level of missing data
6. Consistent delivery of interventions

These features are key because they (1) control error, bias, and unwanted influences; and (2) determine to whom the results will apply. In so doing, they bolster confidence in the credibility and applicability of the findings.

Before explaining these key features, let's consider some of the terminology used in reports of experimental studies. The new intervention (frequently the intervention of greatest interest) may be called the **experimental intervention** or **test intervention**; however, the terms **experimental treatment** and **independent variable** (the cause) is also used. The terms intervention and treatment groups may be used when referring to both interventions. The researcher's control over the design and delivery of the interventions may be referred to as **manipulation of the intervention**. We will use all these terms to help you get accustomed to them.

Research Lingo: Intervention = Treatment = Independent variable

Well-Defined Target Population

When researchers first consider a study, they have a target population in mind. As the study design proceeds, they need to be very clear about the criteria that define the target population, and in so doing they produce a list of **inclusion criteria** (also called *eligibility criteria*). Common inclusion criteria are age range, sex, gender, ethnic group, medical diagnosis, clinical or functional status, care setting, and geographical location. Sometimes, the researcher will specify **exclusion criteria** in addition to inclusion criteria. An example of an exclusion may be persons with physical conditions that would make it inadvisable for them to receive the intervention or participate in the study's requirements. (See example in text box.)

In a study that designed therapeutic play to reduce the stress responses of preschool-aged children hospitalized with an acute respiratory infection, the following eligibility criteria were used:

1. The child age between 3 to 6 years old was admitted to the inpatient hospital with a respiratory infection,
2. The child's parents completed the consent form and agree to participate, and
3. The child verbally agreed to participate.

Children with chronic or critical diseases and/or taking corticosteroids were excluded (Liu & Chou, 2021).

Inclusion and exclusion criteria serve four purposes:

1. Define the population to whom the findings will be generalizable.
2. Identify characteristics that must be present for a person to be included in the sample.
3. Control variables that will distort the results.
4. Make it feasible to conduct the study.

When it is known in advance that a particular patient characteristic strongly influences the outcomes of interest and that characteristic is not of interest in the study, the researcher may decide to remove its influence completely. This is done even though random sampling would even out the variable's influence across the two groups because removing it altogether allows the effect of the treatment being tested to stand out. One way to remove a powerful patient characteristic influence that is not of interest in the study is to include only persons who do not have that characteristic in the study.

To illustrate: If a study of persons with mild congestive heart failure examines the effects of two rehabilitation approaches on the distance they can walk in 6 minutes without stopping to catch their breath or rest, the researcher might exclude persons whose walking is affected by conditions other than their cardiac conditioning. This could be done by excluding all persons with preexisting physical disabilities that affect mobility, such as stroke, severe hip and knee arthritis, peripheral arterial disease, Parkinson's disease, lower-extremity amputation, and neurological disease. From a research point of view, these exclusions make sense in that they control extraneous variables affecting mobility and thereby increase the likelihood that the analysis will identify differences in walking outcomes resulting from the two different rehab approaches. However, a long list of exclusion criteria can also create problems in finding eligible study participants.

From the clinical perspective, many persons with mild congestive heart failure also have arthritis and other mobility conditions. So, a study conducted with this many exclusions would apply only to a very narrow portion of the patients clinicians are likely to see, and we would say the study has limited generalizability in real-world practice. Thus, researchers have to use exclusion criteria with awareness regarding how they will affect the clinical usefulness of the findings.

Adequate Sample Size

An experimental study's sample size must be large enough to differentiate between a true difference and a chance difference in outcomes. A **true difference** is one that is large enough that a difference would likely be found in the population; it is indicated by a significant statistical result (a data-based p-value less than the specified decision point p-level). A **chance difference** is one that just happened in the sample but would probably not be found in the population. Determining "large enough" requires taking the following into account:

1. The expected strength of the experimental intervention's impact vis-à-vis the comparison intervention's impact. The strength of the intervention is often calculated using the smallest difference between groups that would be considered a clinically meaningful impact on patient outcomes.
2. The amount of score dispersion that has been found in prior studies.
3. The desired **level of significance** (i.e., the p-value that will be used as a decision point for **statistical significance**).

These values are entered into a **power analysis** calculation which produces an estimate of the sample size required. You do not need to know how to do a power analysis, but you should know that doing a power analysis is the correct way to determine the sample size for correlational and experimental studies (Gray & Grove, 2021). Power analysis should be done when designing an experimental study to avoid doing a study that has a very low capacity for finding a statistically significant difference in the outcomes of the two groups. Insufficient sample size weakens the capacity of the statistics used to declare a significant difference in the outcomes of the two groups. It is like using a microscope with weak magnification, you know something is there, but it's not clear enough to know if it's something important or not. Researchers use the terms **low statistical power** and **underpowered** to refer to a study with low capacity to declare a significant difference in the outcomes of the two groups. A common reason for low statistical power is a small sample size.

When there is good reason to expect that the intervention will strongly impact the study outcomes, the power analysis usually indicates that a small sample size will be adequate. However, nursing interventions typically have modest impacts. The reality is that many nursing studies done with 30 persons in each group that find no statistically significant difference in the outcomes of the two groups would find one had they been done with 60 or 100 persons in each group. If the purpose of a study is to determine if one intervention is more effective than another, doing a study with too small a sample is a waste of time, effort, and resources on everyone's part (Gray & Grove, 2021).

Random Assignment to Treatment Groups

Random assignment of enrolled participants to treatment groups is a defining feature of experimental studies. It is accomplished by assigning each person in the sample to either the **experimental group** or the comparison group based on chance determination, not on the patient preference for one treatment approach over the other, on physician request, or on the convenience of the research staff. Chance assignment requires that each participant have an equal chance of being assigned to either group. A flip of a coin is one way of randomly assigning each participant to one of the two study groups; more commonly, a computer-generated list of random numbers is used to determine each person's group assignment.

The contribution of random assignment to experimental design is that it controls differences in participant characteristics by distributing them evenly across both treatment groups, thus producing two groups that are similar before the interventions are given. Equivalent groups at the start are necessary in experiments because, at the end of the study, the researcher wants to be confident that different group compositions did not influence the results. When a random assignment is not used, the possibility exists that some difference between the two groups present prior to giving the interventions may have produced the difference found in the outcomes. This possibility creates a lack of confidence that any difference found post-intervention resulted from the interventions they received.

The larger the sample size, the greater the chances that random assignment will create treatment groups equivalent at baseline on important demographic and clinical variables (e.g., age, body mass index, disease severity). Nevertheless, even in large studies, researchers run comparison statistics on important demographic and clinical variables to make sure that random assignment worked effectively. A table profiling the two groups helps answer questions such as:

- Did the groups have similar mean ages?
- Did the groups have approximately equal proportions of men to women?
- Was the health status of the persons in both groups about the same?

In short, random assignment to treatment groups, sometimes referred to as **randomization**, is the most powerful way of ensuring that the two treatment groups are similar at the onset of the study; it works by evening out the presence of participant characteristics across both groups.

However, not all comparisons of treatment effectiveness can use randomization. It may be ethically or practically impossible to randomly assign persons to treatment groups. For instance, comparing the patient outcomes and costs associated with the care of the frail elderly at home with support services versus nursing homes cannot create comparison groups by random assignment of persons to a care setting. The decision regarding how care will be provided to a frail elderly person is highly personal and hinges on many patient, family, and community factors. As a result, the research on this issue would have to use a cohort design (described in Chapter 8).

Random assignment is different from random sampling. Recall that random sampling is a way of obtaining a study sample representative of the target population, whereas random assignment is a way of determining the intervention each study participant will receive; what they share in common is the use of chance to control bias. (Random sampling was discussed in Chapter 5.)

The important point here is that certain patient characteristics can influence the outcomes being studied, thereby complicating comparing the effects of the two treatments. Random assignment controls the influence of patient characteristics by ensuring that the patient characteristics are present to the same extent in both treatment groups.

Having said that, patient characteristics should be approximately equal in both treatment groups. It also should be noted that study designs analyze how patient characteristics affect response to the intervention. These designs (called factorial designs) make important contributions to clinical knowledge because they provide valuable information about persons with whom the intervention is very effective, moderately effective, or ineffective. We will not go there because factorial designs are complex, and describing them here would lead us astray.

Control of Extraneous Variables and Bias

Even when patient characteristics that may influence the outcome variable have been controlled through random assignment, they are still exerting their influence by increasing the variability in the outcome data. This variability makes it more difficult to detect any difference in outcomes between the two groups. To maximize the detection of the relationship between the independent variable and the outcome variable, a potential extraneous variable may be eliminated by exclusion criteria. Thus, exclusion and inclusion criteria control extraneous variables and thereby give prominence to the relationship between the independent and **dependent variables** of the study.

Study activities and the settings in which the study is conducted also give rise to extraneous variables directly influencing the outcome variables. Steps must be taken to **control** them because they mix with the situation and make it difficult to understand the relationship between the interventions and the outcomes. These influences can be persistent across the study setting or can influence one treatment group more than the other.

Sometimes the setting is the larger world of current events. For example, if during the time a study is being conducted to evaluate managing arthritis pain with the use of heat and cold, a new advertisement for a jazzy new whirlpool hits the TV waves big time, the advertisement could influence the results. Some persons in the heat group might be tempted to use the whirlpool instead of heat according to the study protocol. In addition, some of those in the cold group might abandon cold treatment altogether. These changes in participant compliance with their assigned treatment method could result in persons in the treatment groups using different treatments than the study design indicates they are using. If the researcher is monitoring the study setting (immediate and more global), they may be able to detect such an extraneous influence and take steps to moderate it or check out its influence. Researchers develop specific study procedures or protocols to control extraneous variables originating in the study activities. In advance of starting the study, they specify:

- Characteristics of persons who are eligible for the study
- How participants are to be recruited
- How consent to participate in the study will be obtained
- How participants will be randomly assigned to treatment groups
- The activities that compose each treatment
- The conditions under which the treatments will be delivered
- Training of data collectors
- How and when the outcomes will be measured

In studies where a research assistant observes and rates participants' responses, it's too easy for well-intended data collectors to influence the outcome measurement even when they try to be neutral. **Blinding** the data collector controls this source of bias. Blinding is achieved by ensuring that the data collectors do not know which intervention the participant received. Blinding is not always possible. Consider a study comparing the effects of two positioning protocols on the comfort level of persons with fractured hips before surgery. It is almost impossible to blind data collectors as to which intervention the patient is receiving because the patient will be in a position associated with one or the other of the treatments when the data collectors obtain the comfort ratings.

Any important extraneous variable that is not controlled, eliminated, or taken into account statistically becomes a confounding variable; this means that its presence affects the variables being studied so that the results do not reflect the actual relationship between the variables under investigation. In other words, the researcher failed to recognize it, and it was undetected in what was being studied.

Low Level of Missing Data

Another potential source of bias is missing data, also referred to as *lost to follow-up*. This can lead to attrition bias, the unequal loss of participants from different groups in a study. There are a variety of reasons for not having complete data on all participants who were entered into the study and were randomized to a treatment group, including:

- Some participants dropped out of the study (e.g., moved from the area, did not want to continue in the study).

- Some participants' condition worsened so they could not continue in the study (e.g., transferred to ICU, too sick to answer questions).
- Some participants were not available to measure the outcome variable at one or several data collection times (e.g., missed an appointment, could not contribute a specimen).
- The data collector failed to obtain some data (e.g., they were sick, they overlooked something).
- The burden of participating in the study was too great.

Missing data is more of a problem in studies that collect outcome data over weeks, months, or years—in contrast to an intervention being delivered and the outcomes measured just once shortly thereafter. Generally, the reasons for missing data and the pattern of missing data are more important than the amount, although 20% missing data is clearly of more concern than 2% missing data. Also, random missing data is less concerning than a pattern of missing data (Polit & Beck, 2021). Random missing data consists of values missing here and there equally across both study groups. A pattern is present when more data is missing from one group than from the other, or when more data is missing from participants with a certain characteristic, such as the youngest or the oldest.

A high level or a pattern of missing data can change the results of the study because the equivalency between the groups created by randomization is altered. Participants who dropped out of the study might have been different from those who stayed in on an unknown characteristic. This difference might be associated with the outcomes being studied (Stuart et al., 2018). The effect of a high level or pattern of missing data is sometimes difficult to determine. The missing data can make the intervention look more effective than it was or make it look less effective than it was, depending on how those who dropped out are different from those who stayed in the study and how the different characteristic is associated with the study outcomes. A high level or pattern of missing data leaves us wondering: Would the study's outcomes have changed significantly if all persons had completed the study and contributed data?

To illustrate the previous explanation of missing data, consider a hypothetical randomized study evaluating the effectiveness of a smoking cessation method: the study had a larger dropout rate in the test intervention group than in the comparison group. If only data from those who stayed in the study were analyzed, the results may have been biased because only the people who found the test intervention agreeable would be included in the analysis. This would make the test intervention look better than it would have been had all the persons randomized to that group contributed outcome data. The researcher of such a study should ask (1) Why did so many participants drop out of the intervention group? (2) How should I analyze or interpret the data to take this into account?

Because loss to follow-up is a potential source of bias in randomized studies, the CONSORT group (Consolidated Standards of Reporting Trials), a widely recognized organization composed of experts in clinical trial methodology and reporting, addressed loss to follow-up in its guideline for reporting of randomized clinical trials. It recommends that study reports include a flow chart displaying the numbers of study participants from enrollment through data analysis, as shown in **Figure 7-2**.

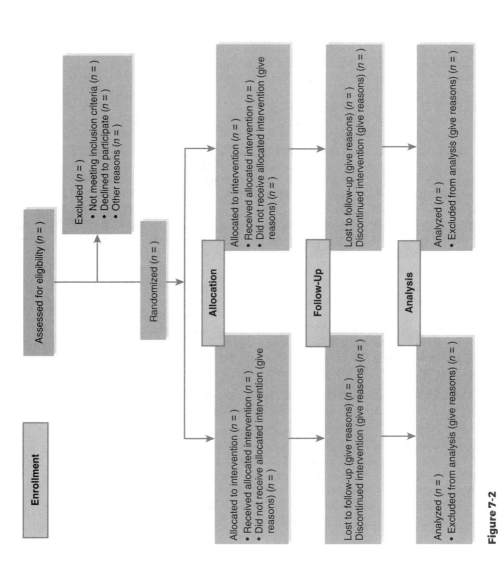

Figure 7-2

Ideally, researchers put in place procedures to reduce the loss of participants during the study, but when it occurs, there are several options: (1) run the data analysis using data only from those with complete data or (2) estimate the missing outcome data using imputation and sensitivity analyses (Nunan et al., 2018). When the first option is used, the researcher must try to understand why the data is missing and what impact it might have had on the results. A rule of thumb states that <5% attrition leads to little bias, while >20% poses serious threats to validity (Nunan et al., 2018). An obvious way is to look at baseline data to see if those who dropped out are in any identifiable way different from those who stayed until study completion. There are several ways of doing the second option, but all involve assumptions about what scores or outcomes the lost-to-follow-up participants might have achieved. For those readers interested in the ways used to estimate values for the missing data, you could look for articles in the health literature about "intention to treat analysis" or "attrition bias."

Large numbers of dropouts and missing data also threaten the generalizability of the study's findings. For example, a randomized study of a new physical activity program for second and third-grade inner-city children might find that the group who participated in the new program did better than those who received a placebo intervention. However, the study had a 26% dropout rate, evenly distributed across both treatment groups. Although the even distribution of dropouts may not have biased the study results, the benefit produced by the new program may not be realized if the program were given to all second and third-grade inner-city kids. The high dropout rate could have produced a study sample that was not representative of the target population, and thus the generalizability of the study findings would be called into question.

While some researchers make a concerted effort to understand the impact of missing data, others, unfortunately, gloss over or ignore it. As a research consumer, you should expect the researcher to acknowledge large amounts or differential loss to follow-up proportions.

Consistent Delivery of Interventions

Two-group experiments involve doing something to half of the participants and something else to the other half. In research language, one group receives the experimental intervention, and the other receives a comparison intervention. The experimental intervention is usually somewhat new in that its effectiveness has not been thoroughly evaluated; however, there should be a good reason to believe that it is safe and will have a meaningful impact on the outcomes of interest. The comparison intervention can take one of five forms (Curtis et al., 2018):

- No intervention at all
- A placebo intervention
- A usual care intervention
- A different intervention
- Same intervention but of different dose (i.e., intensity, frequency, or timing)

Placebo interventions are designed to look and feel similar to the intervention being tested but do not have an effect on the outcomes being studied. At the very least, placebo interventions provide an attention activity for the comparison group to counterbalance the attention the intervention group receives. This is done because the attention involved in delivering an intervention, in and of itself, can impact some outcomes. For this reason, teaching or psychological support intervention studies often use a placebo group rather than a no-intervention group.

The experimental and comparison interventions should be spelt out in considerable detail before starting the study and consistently delivered throughout the study. Steps taken to ensure consistent delivery of the intervention include:

- Specific study protocols
- Training of those who will be delivering the intervention
- Checks on the delivery of the intervention to ensure compliance with study protocols

If either intervention morphs during the study, the contrast between them will be lost. This loss of contrast will invalidate the results because the comparison the researcher set out to make will no longer exist.

Wrap-Up

In summary, an experimental study is usually sound when researchers do the following:

1. Specify the target population
2. Determine sample size by doing a power analysis
3. Use random assignment to ensure that groups are equivalent at the start of the study
4. Control extraneous influences and potential bias
5. Take steps to ensure that participants stay in the study and contribute data at all collection times
6. Ensure that interventions are delivered consistently

Using these research methods ensures that any significant differences detected in the outcomes of the groups studied can be attributed with confidence to the difference in interventions the group received. Furthermore, if no differences are found, the use of these methods ensures that the lack of difference can be attributed to the fact that the two treatments do not have different impacts.

Measurement of the Outcome Variables

As the standard of "good data" (Chapter 5) applies to experimental studies, the instruments used to measure the outcome variables should have high reliability and validity. The researcher should report the reliability and validity testing results that have been done in prior research, particularly testing done in populations similar to the one being studied. Generally speaking, good data is produced by measurement instruments that have been rigorously developed through testing and thus have known reliability and validity levels. Instruments developed for the reported study often lack reliability and validity confirmation because they have no history.

Limitations of Randomized Experiments

The randomized experiment is the gold standard study design for determining if a healthcare intervention brings desired outcomes. However, when clinicians read a study report of a randomized study, they often want to decide if they should use the intervention with their patients; in this regard, randomized studies have limitations. The problem is that many studies' findings are often reported as average outcomes for the two treatment groups. However, clinicians treat unique individuals, not average individuals, and thus the clinician does not know if the particular patient will respond like the average patient in the more effective study group or in a different way. Even if 80% of patients in a group respond favorably to an intervention, the clinician does not know if the patient he is treating will respond like the 80% or the other 20%. One way to address this is to compare the profile of those who responded favorably to those who did not and see if there are any differences.

A second limitation of randomized controlled experiments is that they may have weak generalizability resulting from the exclusion of patients with conditions other than the one of interest as described earlier. Exclusions control extraneous variables and thereby afford more certainty about the effectiveness of the intervention. However, they pose a dilemma for clinicians in that the patients in the study may have fewer health problems (i.e., comorbidities) than patients seen in everyday practice. As a result, the intervention itself may be challenging to use, or similar results may not be realized.

Another issue limiting the generalizability of the findings of randomized controlled experiments is that the interventions are controlled, whereas in everyday practice, an intervention is delivered by a diverse group of clinicians. Often it is not clear how much variation can be introduced into the delivery of an intervention and still retain its effectiveness.

These limitations do not mean that randomized controlled experiments are not useful; however, they do point to the need for multiple studies regarding an intervention under different conditions and with diverse groups of people. The limitations also require that researchers explore deeply why some people responded very positively to an intervention, others responded moderately positively, and others responded negatively or poorly.

Quasi-Experimental Designs

Although the experimental design is the gold standard for evaluating the cause–effect relationship between an intervention and an outcome, sometimes it is *not* possible to (1) use random assignment to intervention groups; (2) have tight control over the delivery of the intervention; or (3) have a comparison group (Gray & Grove, 2021).

Studies that lack one or more of these features are described as **quasi-experimental**. They are enough like experiments to retain the word *experiment* in their description, but because they lack one of the crucial features of experiments, they leave open the door to uncontrolled extraneous variables and wrong conclusions to the extent that experimental designs do not.

To illustrate, if two methods for preventing heel pressure ulcers were studied in a long-term care facility unit, the staff might have difficulty keeping the two methods pure. So, the researchers might decide to use method A with at-risk patients on one unit and method B with at-risk patients on another similar unit. This would be a quasi-experimental study because individual participants are members of intact groups (patients on a particular unit) and the unit determines which intervention they receive, not a random assignment. Even when the two patient groups seem similar, there is concern that they might be different in unidentified ways or that the quality of care in the two units is different. Any difference could act as an extraneous variable giving statistical results indicative of an intervention effect on the outcome when in actuality, it was a patient or unit difference that produced the results, not the intervention. The researcher conducting such a study could take steps to identify, control, or consider extraneous influences. These steps would include comparing the characteristics of the patients in the two units and comparing the two units on variables such as staffing pattern, years of experience of the staff, and their educational levels. Taking any differences into account in the analysis would build confidence in study results indicating that one intervention was more effective than the other in preventing heel ulcers.

Another example of a quasi-experimental design is a study in which the first 100 participants receive treatment A and the second 100 receive treatment B. This would be a consecutive series method for assigning individuals to treatment groups; thus, patient participants are not randomly assigned to treatment groups. This design also raises concerns that the two treatment groups might not be equivalent initially. Something may have changed in the environment during the time that lapsed between the beginning of one series and the beginning of the second series, such as a seasonal difference in patients, a change in staffing, or a change in work flow. Thus, an extraneous variable could be at work and produce a difference in patient outcomes.

Generally, quasi-experimental study designs are considered weaker than randomized experimental designs because there is a lack of certainty that the two groups were equivalent at baseline or received exactly the same treatment. The reader of a report of a quasi-experimental study needs to be alert to nonequivalent groups, inconsistent treatment delivery, or the presence of extraneous variables because they could distort the results and study conclusions.

Exemplar Section 1

Reading Reminder

At this point, read just the *Introduction* and *Material and Methods* sections (up to *Results*) and complete section 1 of your analysis and application table.

Exemplar

Quantitative Experimental Exemplar Article

Erdogan, B., & Aytekin Ozdemir, A. (2021). The effect of three different methods on venipuncture pain and anxiety in children: Distraction cards, virtual reality, and Buzzy® (randomized controlled trial). *Journal of Pediatric Nursing, 58*, e54–e62. https://doi .org/10.1016/j.pedn.2021.01.001

Quantitative Experimental Analysis and Application Table

Section 1		Page
Study Purpose (Why)		
Methods (How)		
Design		
Sample		
Measurement and Quality of Data		
Data Analysis		
Ethics Review		
Section 2		
Results (What)		
Sample and Findings		
Discussion		

Profile & Commentary: Part 1—Why and How

Quantitative Experimental Profile and Commentary on the Exemplar Article

Erdogan, B., & Aytekin Ozdemir, A. (2021). The effect of three different methods on venipuncture pain and anxiety in children: Distraction cards, virtual reality, and Buzzy® (randomized controlled trial). *Journal of Pediatric Nursing, 58,* e54–e62. https://doi.org/10.1016/j.pedn.2021.01.001

Section 1		Page
Study Purpose (Why)	The authors of this study note that the problem is that healthcare professionals managing procedural pain in children do not use many of the studied nonpharmacological and pharmacological interventions because of cost, difficulty to use, or they are time-consuming.	pp. 54–55
	This study, therefore, aimed to determine the effect of Buzzy®, virtual reality, and distraction cards on anxiety and venipuncture pain in children 7–12 years of age.	
	Eight specific research hypotheses are stated. The purpose of this study is straightforward.	
Methods (How)		
Design	The experimental treatments involved randomizing children into four groups: Distraction Cards (DC; n = 35), Virtual Reality (VR; n = 37), Buzzy® (n = 36), and control (n =34). The authors provide a figure of the study flow which clearly lays out sampling.	p. 55
	The control group did not get any nonpharmacological interventions during the routine venipuncture.	p. 58
	Importantly, only one of the blood collection rooms was used for this study, ensuring that each intervention had the same conditions (phlebotomy seat, heat, light, noise, etc.). Also, note that one pediatrician made the decisions, and the venipuncture was completed by the same volunteer nurse with at least 5 years of pediatric venipuncture experience.	p. 58

(continues)

Section 1		Page
Sample	The inclusion and exclusion criteria were detailed. The list of exclusion criteria was fairly long, but understandable in that they excluded children who might have an unusual reaction to the venipuncture and thereby affect the outcomes that were evaluated.	pp. 55–56
	The researchers also considered the following extraneous variables, age, gender, fear of procedure, and controlled for them with block randomization:	p. 55
	Recruitment is not clearly stated; however, based on the inclusion and exclusion criteria we can assume children were recruited if they went to the pediatric venipuncture unit within the hospital and met criteria. We know based on exclusion criteria that the children were not there for a hospital stay, only there for blood tests. However, based on the information provided, we can't determine if the children were having blood tests completed as routine care or for illness. However, the exclusion criteria would seem to limit the sample to basically healthy children.	p. 55
	Sample size—Using G*Power, the researches conducted a power analysis Power analysis should always be done to ensure the study is not underpowered and detect significant differences.	
Measurement and Quality of Data	Before the venipuncture, the researcher collected descriptive characteristics by doing face-to-face interviews. Then, participants were randomly assigned to the groups and along with their parents were informed about the nonpharmacological methods and the scales (VAS, WB-FACES, and CFS). Venipuncture took place either as control group or with assigned nonpharmacological method (distraction cards (DC), virtual reality (VR), and Buzzy®). No pharmacological painkillers were administered before, during, or after venipuncture. The authors clearly state how each group procedure occurred. Following venipuncture, the "participants completed the VAS and WB-FACES (pain levels) and CFS (anxiety levels). Meanwhile, a volunteer parent and the researcher observed the participants' behavior and completed the WB-FACES and CFS."	p. 58

Section 1		Page
	The authors provide information about the reliability and validity of each data collection tool. Of note, they do not strictly state that the tool is reliable and valid, but they provide a good amount of detail on each tool and list references of previous studies that indicate test-retest reliability and construct validity.	pp. 56–58
	Valid and reliable instruments included: 1) The visual analog scale (VAS), 2) Wong-Baker FACES pain rating scale, 3) Children's Fear Scale (CFS), 4) distraction cards, 5) virtual reality, and 6) Buzzy®.	
	All in all, one can conclude that the instruments used in this study have been found to have acceptable reliability and validity.	
Data Analysis	The authors clearly outline the data analysis process. Using the Statistical Package for Social Sciences (SPSS Inc., Chicago, IL, USA) for Windows (version 18.0) the data was analyzed. Statistical significance level was set at 0.05. Distributions, means, chi-square tests, and standard deviations were used for analysis. Levene's test and a post-hoc Bonferroni was used for further analysis.	p. 58
Ethics Review	Ethical considerations were noted. The researcher's ethics committee approved the study at their institution. The study's purpose and procedures were provided to participants and their parents, obtaining signed informed consent from the parents and verbal consent from the children. Participants had the right, without any explanation, to withdraw from the study at any time.	p. 56
	As this study involved collecting data from children, there may have been special conditions that had to be met for approval by the ethical commission. In the United States, when children age 7 or older are involved in research, IRBs generally require the assent of the child as well as the written permission of the parent(s). The child's assent is required when the child has the capacity to comprehend what the study will require of them; parents must give permission before the researcher contacts the child for assent (U.S. Department of Health and Human Services, n.d.).	

(continues)

Section 1		Page
	In this study, having venipuncture was not a research variable as all participants part of inclusion criteria required blood tests. So, the study itself did not do anything to the child that was hurtful, invasive, or risky and imposed only a very low burden of effort on child and parent. Thus, it was a low-risk study. We don't know exactly how all this was handled, but the authors inform us that before venipuncture the participants and parents were informed about the nonpharmacological methods and the scales. Having a procedure and script, it undoubtedly required or was at least reviewed by the Ethical Commission.	

Section 2: Study Results

More Effective?

In most two-group experimental studies, the researcher's goal is to determine if one intervention is more effective. Effectiveness is the impact or influence on the outcome variable(s), and more effective is a greater degree of positive impact or influence. There are two ways of thinking about effectiveness: from the clinical and statistical perspectives. At the center of both perspectives is a comparison of the size of the effect each intervention had on the outcome variable of the two groups. From the clinical perspective, the bottom-line question is, "Is the difference in the outcomes of the two groups large enough to be clinically meaningful to patients or how I practice?" This perspective on the data is referred to as the *importance* or *practical significance* of the results. From the statistical perspective, the bottom-line question is, "Is the difference found a true difference that is likely in the target population or a chance difference unique to this sample?" When reading a report of an intervention study, too many people get hung up in the results of the statistical analysis (e.g., *p*-values, statistical significance). We suggest you start by first considering the results from a clinical perspective and then proceed to consider the meaning of the statistical tests of significance.

Generally speaking, the results of 2-group experimental studies are reported in one of two ways:

1. As the mean scores of the two groups on the outcome variable
2. As the percentage of persons in each group who achieved a clinical outcome or milestone

Some studies report mean scores and no percentages attaining particular clinical outcomes, whereas other studies report attainment of clinical outcome attainment percentages and no mean scores. A few studies report both.

Outcome Reported as a Mean

When the outcome variable of a study is measured on an interval-level scale, a score is obtained for every patient, and group means and/or medians are calculated for the control and intervention groups. The term *score* refers to the numerical values obtained by all measurement forms, physiological measurements, questionnaires, or rating scales. The explanations below will focus on means, although the general principles could also be applied to medians, the other measure of central tendency. If you are unsure when medians are used instead of means and the inferential tests used in analyzing them, you should consult a statistics book.

Clinical Perspective on Mean Differences

To make clinical sense of the results, you should first note the difference between the means of the two groups by subtracting one from the other—keeping in mind the range of the scale that was used to measure the variable. Then ask: Is this difference large enough to have clinical importance? For example:

- Is a mean difference of 950 cc per day between the mean fluid intakes of two groups large enough to make a difference in patients' hydration status?
- Is a mean 8 mm difference between the two groups' mean diastolic blood pressure levels large enough to represent better blood pressure control and lowered risk of complications?

Considering the size of the difference between the means of the two groups provides some clinical sense of whether the difference in the impact of the two treatments is large, small, or somewhere in between. The size of the difference is a point estimate based on the sample, and the difference found in the population could be somewhat lower or higher. If the researcher provides a confidence interval (**Figure 7-3**) around the difference in the means, that will give you a better sense of the high and low that might be realized in the target population (Gray & Grove, 2021).

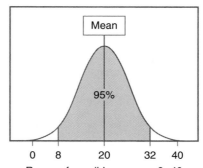

Range of possible scores = 0–40
Mean difference found in study = 20
Likely difference in target population = 8–32

Figure 7-3 95% Confidence Interval

The takeaway: Considering the difference in means between the two groups from a clinical/practical perspective is a valuable starting point for making practical sense of results.

Statistical Perspective on Mean Differences

When an outcome variable of a study is measured on an interval level scale, and the results are reported as the means of each group, the statistical analysis provides valuable information in answering the question: *Is the difference between the* means *of the two groups a true difference or a chance difference?* A true difference between the mean scores of the two groups is a difference that is robust enough that a difference is also likely to occur in the target population, not just in the study sample; the difference found in the population could be higher or lower than what was found in the study, but it is likely a difference will be found. A chance difference is caused by the normal variation in outcomes one would expect when measuring an outcome in two samples drawn from the same population; it is unlikely that a difference would be found in the target population.

In an experimental study, the two groups received different treatments; therefore, a difference in outcome scores is of interest. A treatment effect is present when one treatment produces a larger effect on the outcome than the other. The larger the difference found between the outcome mean of the two groups, the greater the chance that the difference is caused by one group receiving a truly more effective treatment. Moreover, the larger the difference in the means of the two groups, the greater the likelihood that a difference would be found if the whole target population had been studied.

Note that your starting point is common sense, even for the statistical question. Sometimes, by looking at the outcome mean scores of the two groups and noting how different or close they are, you can get a first impression regarding whether the difference is caused by treatment effect or is just **chance variation**. However, the definitive answer regarding whether the difference is a true difference or a chance difference is provided by inferential statistics. In comparing the scores of two groups with interval-level outcome data, the *p*-value result produced by a *t*-test provides the definitive answer regarding the interpretation of a difference in group mean scores. (Note that different statistics are used when the outcome data is reported as group median scores.).

> The *t*-test results provide the definitive answer regarding whether a difference in mean effectiveness is likely in the target population.

t-*Test and* p-*Value*

The ***t*-test** is used to compare scores of two groups when the outcome variable is measured using an interval level scale, and the mean is the average being analyzed; it should not be used when the data are skewed or when the outcome variable is a proportion or a categorical variable. The ***t*-test** analyzes the size of the difference between the means of two groups while taking into account the sample size and the spread of the scores across the possible range of scores (i.e., the standard deviation). It essentially asks: Even though a difference in means was found in this sample, what are the chances that *no* difference would be found in the target population?

The *t*-test analysis produces a *p*-value indicating the probability that the difference found between the means is just a chance occurrence. This data-based *p*-value probability is compared to a previously chosen level of significance *p*-level decision point. A *p*-value at or lower than the decision point represents a low probability that the difference found is just a chance difference; a *p*-value higher than the decision point represents high levels of risk that the difference found is a chance difference. Thus, if the data-based *p*-value is equal to or lower than the decision point *p*-level, the researcher will conclude that the difference found is true; i.e., a difference would likely be found in the population and in this sample. In contrast, if the data-based *p*-value is higher than the decision point *p*-level, the researcher will conclude that the difference found is a chance difference, i.e., no difference is likely to occur in the population.

The researcher does not want to wrongly conclude that a difference is a true difference when in reality, it is a chance difference; by only accepting a low level of probability that the difference is a chance difference, they can be quite confident when saying, "This is a true difference." Often, but not always, the level of significance decision point is set at 0.05. By setting it there, the researcher accepts a 5% or less risk of being wrong when they say the difference found is true.

So, let's say the researcher set the level of significance decision point at $p = 0.05$, and the data-based *p*-value comes in at 0.03. The researcher had decided in advance that they would be willing to accept a 5% chance of being wrong when concluding that the difference found is not just a chance occurrence, and the result of $p = 0.03$ indicates there is just a 3% chance that they would be wrong. So, the researcher says, "Okay, I'm confident in concluding that the difference found between the two groups is a true difference. I conclude because there is only a 3% chance that I am wrong." In research lingo, a result like this would be reported: "The difference found was statistically significant at the $p \leq 0.05$ level."

In contrast, consider the situation in which the researcher also sets the level of significant decision point at $p = 0.05$, but the data-based *p*-value comes in at 0.08. This result means that the researcher was willing to accept a 5% chance of being wrong when concluding that the difference found was a true difference, but the difference found results in an 8% chance that they would be wrong in concluding that the difference found is a true difference. In this situation, the researcher will think, "If I conclude this is a true difference, there is too high a probability of being wrong. Therefore, I will conclude that the difference found could be a chance occurrence, and no difference would likely be found in the population." A result like this would be reported as not significant (ns). The contrasting types of statistical results just described are portrayed graphically in **Figure 7-4**. Hopefully, it will make these complex issues clearer.

Scenario

A hypothetical study tested the effects of two different methods of reducing discomfort in adults while freezing a precancerous lesion on the lower leg with liquid nitrogen (method A and method B); the person's pain experience during the freezing was determined immediately after the procedure using a scale with a

Data-based p-value	< .001	.01	.025	**.05**	.08	.15	.59 >
Finding	Significant difference				Not significant difference		
Conclusion	A difference would likely be found in the population.				A difference would *not* likely be found in the population.		

*Using a .05 level of significance decision point

Figure 7-4 Interpretation of p-Values Produced by t-Tests

value range of 0 to 10 (0 being no pain, 10 being a great deal of pain). Group A ($n = 42$) had a mean score of 3.6 and group B ($n = 40$) had a mean of 4.6, indicating that those in the method A group had on average less pain. A t-test was run on the difference between the means (1 point), and the result was $p = 0.02$. This is the data-based probability value; it indicates there are only 2 chances in 100 that a difference this large would occur because of chance variation. Said differently, if the researcher concluded that method A was more effective than method B, there would be 2 chances in 100 that his or her conclusion is wrong. When this data-based probability is compared to the decision point level of significance probability ($p = 0.05$), the conclusion would be that it is a true difference in outcome, because there is an acceptably low probability that the difference is just chance variation. See the Scenario 1 summary in **Table 7-1**.

Consider a different result for this study: Group A had a mean of 3.6, group B had a mean of 3.8, and $p = 0.14$ (Scenario 2 in Table 7-1). Now, the difference is just 0.2 and there are 14 chances in 100 that the difference was a chance result. With this result, *if* the researcher concluded that the difference is true, there would be 14 chances in 100 that his conclusion would be wrong. Based on the researcher's chosen level of significant decision point ($p \leq 0.05$), this is too high a chance of being wrong, so the researcher would conclude the two methods of comforting are essentially equivalent; i.e., a difference in effectiveness is doubtful, the difference found is not significant.

Summary of p-Values

A difference in means associated with a low p-value (i.e., a data-based p-value equal to or below the decision point p-level) is considered statistically significant; it is a true difference in treatment effectiveness, meaning that a difference would likely be found in the population as well. A difference with a high p-value (i.e., a data-based p-value above the decision point p-level) is considered not significant, meaning the probability that it is a chance difference is high; a difference would most likely not be found in the population. In study reports, the statistics just described are reported in various ways. The absolute difference between the means of the two groups' outcomes may or may not be stated, but it can be easily calculated by

Table 7-1 Statistical Conclusions

Scenario 1	Group A	Group B	
Mean pain level	3.6	4.6	
Difference in the means	1		
Level of significance p-level			0.05
Data-based $p =$			0.02
Conclusion			True difference
Probability that conclusion is wrong			2%
Scenario 2	**Group A**	**Group B**	
Mean pain level	3.6	3.8	
Difference in the means		.2	
Level of significance p-level			0.05
Data-based $p =$			0.14
Conclusion			Chance difference
Probability that conclusion is wrong			Not easily calculated

subtracting one group's mean from the other's mean. The *t*-value may or may not be reported, but in and of itself, it is not of importance to the clinical reader. However, the *p*-value associated with a *t*-test or an indication of whether the difference is statistically significant will almost always be provided in the text or indicated by a symbol in a table.

Reporting of p-Values

Researchers aim to present their results in both honest and favorable ways. For that reason, you will see a variety of adjectives used to describe the significance of results. When the researcher preset the significance level *p*-level at 0.05 and the data-based *p*-value comes in at 0.02 or 0.03, the researcher may connote this with a symbol or superscript letter indicating that the result was *significant at* $p \leq 0.05$. However, if the data-based *p*-value came in at 0.002, the researcher may describe the result as *highly significant*. This communicates that there is an even lower probability of the difference found being a chance event—much lower than the decision point they had set—thus they are very confident that the difference found is a true difference.

Another scenario is that the data-based *p*-value is just above the decision point *p*-level, $p = 0.06$ or 0.07. The researcher might say that the result was "marginally

---

Box 7-1 Example of *p*-Value Interpretation

In a randomized controlled trial of the efficacy of a breathing training program on depression in patients on hemodialysis (Tsai et al., 2015), the participants who received breathing training showed a mean reduction 3.69 points on their depression score whereas the control group had a 1.48 mean reduction. The difference was significant at the $p = 0.01$ level. Thus, there is just 1 chance in 100 that a difference in depression would not be found in the larger population.

---

significant" or "approached significance." This conveys that the *p*-value was close to the level of significance decision point; i.e., the difference in the two means was almost large enough to have confidence that it is a true difference. Reporting marginal results is justified when the study is an early test of an intervention because it may indicate a promising intervention that warrants another study.

Did we lose you in the last six to eight pages? If so, you need to go back to your statistics book and read about hypothesis testing, the *t*-test, and *p*-values. We offer the observation that the meaning of *p*-values will become clearer as you read more study reports. You will, however, have to pay attention to the *p*-values provided in reports and note how the researchers interpret them. This way, your understanding of them will increase over time. Understanding the meaning of *p*-values is crucial to understanding reports of quantitative studies. It is a concept that you must master.

Attainment of an Outcome

When attainment of an outcome or milestone is reported as a "yes" or "no," it is called a dichotomous outcome. Examples of **dichotomous variables** are these:

- Complication/no complication
- Increased self-care knowledge/did not increase self-care knowledge
- Gained the ability to walk 50 feet without assistance/did not gain this ability
- Smoking at 1 year after intervention/not smoking at 1 year

Clinical Perspective on Proportions

In experimental studies with dichotomous outcomes, the proportions of persons in each treatment group who attained the yes/no outcomes are determined. You can look at the two proportions and determine whether the difference in proportions is large or small. This difference can be clarified further. When an outcome is a good event, the difference in these two proportions is called the **absolute benefit increase (ABI)**. It is one of several measures of treatment effect used to portray the relative impact of two treatments (Gray & Grove, 2021). The other one explained next is the **number needed to treat (NNT)**.

Let's start with a concrete example: a study in which a new program to encourage physical activity in second- and third-grade inner-city kids is evaluated. (Focus on the results, not the study design, and assume a low rate of dropout.) Two hundred children were randomly assigned to attend the new once-a-week after-school exercise program for 3 weeks or to receive a placebo treatment in which a study assistant played electronic, card, and board games with them once a week for 3 weeks.

The milestone outcome being considered is actively exercising for 8 hours or more outside of school each week when measured 3 months after the program; this is a dichotomous outcome that is either achieved or not achieved. The results showed that 26% of the kids in the program attained the milestone outcome, whereas 12% of those in the placebo group attained it; stated as proportions, these percentages are 0.26 and 0.12. So, the difference between the proportion of those in the program who met the milestone and the proportion in the placebo group who met it is 0.14 (0.26 minus 0.12); thus, the ABI produced by the exercise intervention over the placebo intervention is 14%. The clinical ramifications of this measure of clinical significance should be considered: Is this a sizable enough difference to justify saying that the new program has a success rate that is clinically important?

The NNT provides an even better take on this question. It is the number of kids who would have to be given the more effective treatment rather than the less effective treatment for one additional kid to achieve the milestone outcome. In our fictional study, the NNT is 8. This means that for every eight kids entered into the exercise program, rather than just getting attention, one kid will achieve the milestone exercise level who would not have had s/he they just received attention. This provides a practical sense of how much benefit the exercise program would produce over just attention. Note that the NNT is easily calculated from the ABI; it is the inverse (reciprocal) of the ABI. That is, 1/ABI rounded up to a whole number—we do not treat 0.1 of a person. These measures of benefit are portrayed in **Table 7-2**.

NNT is helpful for two reasons. First, it provides a clinical perspective on how many more people are likely to benefit at a meaningful level from the exercise program compared with no program. If the NNT were 3 or 4, it would mean that the exercise program is very effective, whereas an NNT of 20 or 30 would mean that quite a few would have to receive it for one additional person to benefit. Second, NNT can be considered in the context of the cost of the program, risks of exercise, and long-term risks of not developing an exercise habit. Combining NNT, the costs of implementing the program and the costs of the kids not developing an exercise habit, the NNT of 8 benefit could be a good value.

Statistical Perspective on Proportions

Researchers often want to know whether the difference in the proportions that attained the clinical outcomes in the two groups is large enough to be likely in the larger population, so they will run a chi-square statistical test or a binomial test. These statistical tests produce a *p*-value indicating whether the difference in the

Table 7-2 Exercise Program for Kids: Measures of Clinical Effect

Measures of Clinical Effect (dichotomous data)	
Milestone attained with program	26% (0.26)
Milestone attained without program	12% (0.12)
Absolute benefit increase (ABI)	14% (0.14)
Number needed to treat (NNT)	$1 \div .14 = 7.1$ rounded up to 8

proportion in the two groups is large enough to be statistically significant, i.e., a difference in proportions between the two groups would be likely in the population. Thus, the data-based p-value of these tests is interpreted in the same way as the t-test's p result, even though the data consisted of proportions and a different statistical test was run.

Example of p-Value for a Difference in Proportions

Two strategies for teaching inhaler use during discharge from acute care hospitals were compared; the control group received a brief intervention, and written instruction and the other group received teach-to-goal education, also known as teach-back (Press et al., 2016). Patients who received teach-to-goal education were less likely to report having required acute care at 30 days compared with the brief instruction group (17% vs. 36%; $p = .03$) but there was no significant difference at 90 days (34% vs. 38%, $p = 0.6$). (Note that the latter p-value is 0.6, not 0.06.) The researchers concluded that teach-to-goal has short-term benefits, but ongoing instruction regarding inhaler technique is required to achieve long-term skill retention and improved health outcomes.

Both Perspectives

Having explained both the clinical perspective and the statistical perspective for both types of study results, we want to point out that statistical significance and clinical significance do not necessarily equate; rather, their relationship can take different forms:

1. The difference between the outcomes of the two treatment groups can be *clinically significant* and *statistically significant*. This would occur when the difference between means is large—of course, large is relative to the nature of the outcome being studied and to the scale used to measure it.
2. The difference can be *clinically not significant* and *statistically not significant*. This would occur when the difference between the means of the two groups is very small.
3. The difference between the two groups can be *clinically significant* but *statistically insignificant*. This occurs most frequently in studies with small sample sizes, which are common in nursing. The clinician sees promise in the results, even though statistically, they could be due to chance, and believes that the intervention needs to be studied with a larger sample.
4. The difference between two group means can be *clinically not significant* but *statistically significant*; from a practical clinical perspective, it is trivial or unimportant. Statistically significant but clinically not significant results frequently occur in studies with very large sample sizes.

Possible Result Combinations

- Clinically significant and statistically significant CS-SS
- Clinically not significant and statistically not significant Cs-Ss
- Clinically significant and statistically not significant CS-Ss
- Clinically not significant and statistically significant Cs-SS

Table 7-3 Weight Loss Example

	New Program Group *n* = 50	Old Program Group *n* = 50
Mean lb lost at 6 months	13 lbs (sd = 4.9)	10.6 lbs (5.3)
Difference in the two means = 2.4 lbs		
95% Cl of the difference: 0.37 to 4.4 lbs		
t-test *p*-value: 0.02		
% achieved a 10 lb loss or more	52%	30%

ABI = 22% NNT = 5 (1 ÷ 0.22 = 4.5 rounded up)

The results of a fictional randomized study comparing a new weight loss program to a program that has been around for a while are displayed in **Table 7-3**. First, note that the two groups' mean difference in weight loss is 2.4 pounds and is statistically significant ($p = 0.02$). Nevertheless, do you think it is clinically significant? Note that the ABI and the NNT are more impressive than the mean difference. Based on the NNT of 5 for a weight loss of 10 pounds or more, we are inclined to say that the new program achieves a weight loss clinically significant for more people than the old program. However, this is an opinion, and others may look at these results and say that the effectiveness of the two programs is not different enough to make a meaningful change in weight over time. Ultimately, this call must be made with the details of the full report and within the context of participants' feelings about the demands and cost of the two programs.

In many nursing studies, consideration of the clinical significance of the difference between outcomes is as important, if not more important, than consideration of whether the results are statistically significant. Unfortunately, the size of the clinical impact of the better intervention is not always discussed in a useful way in reports of nursing intervention studies—even though it should be. Once again, we would advise you not to obsess over the statistical results in a report; instead, think about the size of the difference between the outcomes of the two groups from a clinical perspective before moving on to thinking about them from the statistical perspective.

Opinion Regarding Reporting of Outcomes

Dichotomous (attained or didn't attain) clinical outcomes and their associated measures of effectiveness, ABI and NNT, are widely reported in the medical research literature but less often in the nursing literature. Hopefully, reporting dichotomous clinical outcomes will increase nursing research because they add relevancy for clinicians. This is so because attaining clinical outcomes and milestones is often important to patients—and memorable for clinicians. In contrast, mean scores on a scale or test are often indirect measures of outcomes important to patients and clinicians. We believe that reporting the attainment of dichotomous patient outcomes adds clarity and clinical relevance to study reports.

Consider a fictional study of persons facing a risky medical procedure who were taught different ways of controlling anxiety in the days prior to the procedure; anxiety was measured on the morning of the procedure using a scale in which a low score indicated low anxiety and a high score indicated high anxiety. If the results reveal that the group taught method A had a mean anxiety score of 3 and group taught method B had a mean anxiety score of 7, we could say that clearly method A produced better anxiety prevention/relief. However, we do not get a practical sense of how using method A improved patients' anxiety experiences. In contrast, if the results were reported as 11% of the persons in group A reported enough anxiety that it interfered with their sleep during one of the two nights before surgery and 24% of those in group B reported sleep disturbance during those nights, the difference in treatment effectiveness has immediate clinical relevance.

Exemplar Section 2

Reading Reminder

At this point, you read the *Introduction* and *Material and Methods* sections (up to *Results*) and completed section 1 of your analysis and application table. Now you will read the *Results and Discussion* sections of the exemplar study and complete section 2 of your analysis and application table.

Section 2		Page
Results (What)	The results are reported in the text and in the three tables provided. Focus on the tables. Note that in Table 2, the five outcomes—children's VAS, WB-FACES and CFS scores, parents' report, and researcher report—are measured on interval level scales and reported as means plus standard deviations and *p*-values.	pp. 58–59
Sample and Findings	Comparison of groups preintervention: In Table 1, the four groups are profiled. From it we learn that randomization created four very similar treatment groups because of all the variables (age, gender, fear of venipuncture). The difference between the groups is small and the data-based *p*-values for the differences are high. Thus, the differences are just chance variation that one would expect in drawing four samples from the same population. It is important that we know that the fear of venipuncture levels of the four groups are essentially equal because this variable could be extraneous if it were not equal in all groups.	

Section 2		Page
	Comparison of procedural pain and anxiety scores of the study groups:	
	In Table 2, we see how the children scored the pain and anxiety they experienced during the procedure. First, the mean scoring of the parent and the observer are quite close together, which supports the validity of the measures used. From the clinical perspective, comparing the mean values of the groups on both the WB-FACES (1 to 10) and the VAS (0 to 10), we see there is quite a difference between groups (almost 3 points on the WB-FACES and about 3 points on the VAS). From the statistical perspective, the far-right columns tell us that the analysis indicates that there is essentially no chance ($p < 0.001$) that the differences between the groups could just be due to chance; rather they are different because the groups received different pain interventions—with the Buzzy group followed by the VR, DC, and control groups reporting significantly lower pain and anxiety. Thus, a difference in the target population would likely occur under similar conditions.	p. 59
	Pairwise comparisons of the study groups:	p. 59
	In Table 3 we further see the significant differences between groups. Statistical significance in pain between the DC and Buzzy® groups ($p < 0.05$). Also, statistical significance in anxiety between the DC and Buzzy® groups ($p < 0.05$). From a statistical perspective, the significant differences indicate that the differences are not chance; rather, they are inferred to be the result of receiving the pain intervention or not.	pp. 59 –60
Discussion	Limitations:	p. 61
	The authors acknowledge limitations of their study: 1)The authors acknowledge that the researcher randomized the participants, therefore was not double-blinded; however, to reduce bias, more than one rater scored the anxiety and pain levels; the researcher, participants, and their parents were not blinded to anxiety and pain assessment; 3) the small sample size limits generalizability of venipuncture procedures.	

References

Curtis, M. J., Alexander, S., Cirino, G., Docherty, J. R., George, C. H., Giembycz, M. A., Hoyer, D., Insel, P. A., Izzo, A. A., Ji, Y., MacEwan, D. J., Sobey, C. G., Stanford, S. C., Teixeira, M. M., Wonnacott, S., & Ahluwalia, A. (2018). Experimental design and analysis and their reporting II: Updated and simplified guidance for authors and peer reviewers. *British Journal of Pharmacology, 175*(7), 987–993. https://doi.org/10.1111/bph.14153

Erdogan, B., & Aytekin Ozdemir, A. (2021). The effect of three different methods on venipuncture pain and anxiety in children: Distraction cards, virtual reality, and Buzzy® (randomized controlled trial). *Journal of Pediatric Nursing, 58*, e54–e62. https://doi.org/10.1016/j.pedn.2021.01.001

Gray, J. R., & Grove, S. K. (2021). *Burns and Grove's The practice of nursing research: Appraisal, synthesis, and generation of evidence* (9th ed.). Elsevier Saunders.

Liu, M. C., & Chou, F.-H. (2021). Play effects on hospitalized children with acute respiratory infection: An experimental design study. *Biological Research for Nursing, 23*(3), 430–441. https://doi.org/10.1177/1099800420977699

Nunan, D., Aronson, J., & Bankhead, C. (2018). Catalogue of bias: Attrition bias. *BMJ Evidence-Based Medicine, 23*(1), 21–22. https://doi.org/10.1136/ebmed-2017-110883

Polit, D. F., & Beck, C. T. (2021). *Essentials of nursing research: Appraising evidence for nursing practice* (10th ed.). Lippincott Williams & Wilkins.

Press, V., Arora, V. M., Trela, K. C., Adhikari, R., Zadravecz, F. J., Liao, C., et al. (2016). Effectiveness of interventions to teach metered-dose and diskus inhaler techniques: A randomized trial. *Annals of the American Thoracic Surgery Society, 13*(6), 816–824. https://doi.org/10.1513/AnnalsATS.201509-603OC

Stuart, E. A., Ackerman, B., & Westreich, D. (2018). Generalizability of randomized trial results to target populations: Design and analysis possibilities. *Research on Social Work Practice, 28*(5), 532–537. https://doi.org/10.1177/1049731517720730

U.S. Department of Health and Human Services. (n.d.). *Research with children FAQs*. https://www.hhs.gov/ohrp/regulations-and-policy/guidance/faq/children-research/index.html

variables could have influenced the occurrence of the outcomes of interest. This combination of analyses allows the researcher to:

1. Compare the risk of two groups for the outcomes of interest
2. Determine whether the risks of the two groups are significantly different
3. Check for the effect of possible confounding variables

Reading Tip: You might want to reread the logistic regression and odds ratio sections in Chapter 6 under the *More Complex Designs* section heading.

Confounding

The primary concern in cohort studies is that the two groups could be different in some way other than the presence or absence of the risk factor, and that difference may produce different outcomes for the two groups. For instance, they may have different biophysical characteristics, lifestyles, or experiences. The difference could be something as easy to identify as an age difference or something more difficult to identify, such as different levels of nutrition during youth. If the difference is a determinant of the outcomes being studied and is unequally distributed in the two groups, it is called a **confounding variable** (D'Andrea et al., 2021). Recognizing confounders in advance of a study allows researchers to collect data about them and run analyses to check on their influence on the outcome variable. In the exemplar study for this chapter, you will learn about the techniques researchers take to rule out confounding variables. However, even when the analysis has ruled out suspected confounders, cohort studies are still vulnerable to unknown confounders.

Other Limitations

Cohort studies that follow participants for long periods often suffer from high dropout rates. High dropout rates can bias the incidence of the outcome in either or both groups, thus confounding the results. Another limitation of cohort design is that it does not work well if the outcome being studied occurs rarely. A rare outcome would require following a very large number of people to detect a connection between the risk factor and the outcome. Therefore, when the outcome being studied is rare, researchers may use another design: case-control design.

Case-Control Studies

In a sense, a **case-control study** is the opposite of a cohort study. Remember, a cohort study starts retrospectively or prospectively identifying cohorts of persons to determine if they developed or will develop specific outcomes. A case-control study is a retrospective design that clearly defines the two groups at the start: one with the outcome/disease and one without the outcome/disease. Case-control studies retrospectively assess whether there is a statistically significant difference in the rates of exposure to a defined risk factor between the groups. Retrospective cohort studies are **not** the same as case-control studies. In retrospective cohort studies, the exposure and outcomes have already happened. The logistics of the two types of studies are shown in **Figure 8-1**.

Cohort study

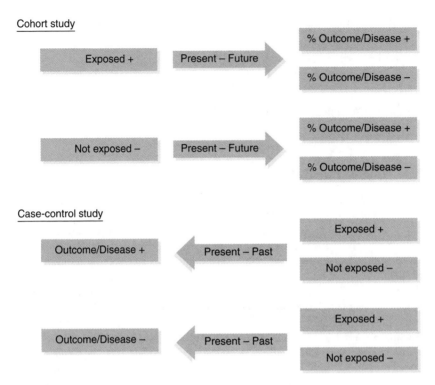

Figure 8-1 Cohort Study vis-à-vis Case-Control Study

Generally, cohort studies are used to study exposures and outcomes that occur relatively frequently and outcomes that develop or occur not too long after the risk factor or exposure. In contrast, case-control studies are used to study outcomes that are rare or take a long time to become evident (e.g., osteoporosis fracture, lung cancer). Case-control studies are even more prone to confounding by unknown factors than cohort studies. They are highly prone to confounding variables because the study involves looking back in time, and important data may not be available or forgotten or distorted by memory.

For example, a case-control study was conducted to determine the association of Chorangiosis with pregnancy complications and perinatal outcomes. "Chorangiosis is a vascular change involving the terminal chorionic villi in the placenta. It results from longstanding, low-grade hypoxia in the placental tissue and is associated with such conditions as intrauterine growth restriction (IUGR), diabetes, and gestational hypertension in pregnancy. Chorangiosis rarely occurs in normal pregnancies. However, its prevalence is 5–7% of all placentas from infants admitted to newborn intensive care units" (Vafaei et al., 2021, Abstract). During a 4-year period, April 2014 to March 2018, 308 cases diagnosed with Chorangiosis matched with 308 other placenta complications were identified. Maternal, placental, prenatal, and neonatal features of the participants were retrospectively derived from the medical records of mothers whose placentas had been sent to the pathology department. Potential confounding effects of maternal age, gestational age, gravid, and parity were controlled by adjusted regression tests in the analysis phase. Thus, by retrospectively looking at Chorangiosis and other placenta complications, this case-control study concluded that although

Chorangiosis is an uncommon condition, it is associated with a higher incidence of perinatal and neonatal morbidity and mortality (Vafaei et al., 2021).

Wrap-Up

Cohort studies provide a way of evaluating risk factors for health conditions or events; they do so by comparing groups with and without exposure to a pre-identified risk factor. Because random assignment is not used to form the comparison groups, cohort studies are prone to confounding variables, threatening the validity of study conclusions about the relationship between the risk factor and the outcome of interest. However, cohort studies provide control over follow-up and diagnosis of the outcome. An alternative design that is used to study risk factors when the outcome of interest is rare is the case-control study, but this design has even more tremendous potential for confounding variables.

Exemplar

Quantitative Cohort Exemplar Article

Ma, J., Li, C., Zhang, W., Zhou, L., Shu, S., Wang, S., Wang, D., & Chai, X. (2021). Preoperative anxiety predicted the incidence of postoperative delirium in patients undergoing total hip arthroplasty: A prospective cohort study. *BMC Anesthesiology, 21*(1), **Article 48. https://doi.org/10.1186/s12871-021-01271-3.**

Quantitative Cohort Analysis and Application Table

		Page
Study Purpose (Why)		
Methods (How)		
Design		

(continues)

		Page
Sample		
Measurement and Quality of Data	**Interrater Reliability**	
Data Analysis		
Ethics Review		
Results (What)		
Sample		
Findings		
Discussion		

Quantitative Cohort Profile and Commentary on the Exemplar Article

Data from Ma, J., Li, C., Zhang, W., Zhou, L., Shu, S., Wang, S., Wang, D., & Chai, X. (2021). Preoperative anxiety predicted the incidence of postoperative delirium in patients undergoing total hip arthroplasty: A prospective cohort study. *BMC Anesthesiology,* *21*, Article 48. https://doi.org/10.1186/s12871-021-01271-3. This article is published under a CC-BY Creative Common License https://creativecommons.org/licenses/by/4.0

		Page
Study Purpose (Why)	This study was conducted to investigate the effect of preoperative anxiety on postoperative delirium.	Abstract
	This prospective study was developed to clarify the relationship between the postoperative anxiety (POA) and the postoperative delirium (POD) via orthopedic surgery. The aim of the study was to investigate whether the POA would predict the onset of POD in patients undergoing the total hip arthroplasty (THA).	p. 2
	In terms of a cohort study, then:	
	Population: Persons having THA	
	Risk cohorts: Anxiety and non-anxiety— note the definition of anxiety, scale used (HADS-A) and this exemplar study Figure 1 Flow of participants in the trial	pp. 2–3
	Outcome variables: POD in THA patients— note the definition of delirium and scale used (CAM)	
Methods (How)		
Design	The design of this study was a prospective cohort design. Prospective indicates that the participants were entered into the study and followed to determine how many developed POD after THA.	p. 2
	Risk Factor of Interest	
	Prior research indicates that POD, defined as a sudden onset of disturbances in attention, consciousness, and other cognitive abilities, is one of the common surgical complications with bad outcomes. The underlying pathogenesis mechanism of delirium the many risk factors,	

(continues)

		Page
	reported by previous studies, for delirium, but POA was of great significance to this study for identifying the relationship of POA and POD because it was unclear and needed further clarification. Also, note orthopedic surgery, especially hip surgery in the elderly was targeted because this population has a higher incidence of POD. Many cohort studies rely on patient reports and medical records regarding exposure to the risk factor. This study collected information about participant demographics and clinical characteristics from the clinical medical chart.	
Sample	The target population was people aged 18 years or older, ASA I-III, undergoing the THA at the Anhui Provincial Hospital (AHPH) from October 2019 to May 2020. Individuals were excluded if they (1) were unable to provide written informed consent, (2) were not fluent in Chinese, (3) had a history of depression or diagnosed with depression (assessed with the Hospital Anxiety and Depression Scale-Depression and diagnosed by psychiatrists), (4) had dementia or scored 24 or lower on the Mini-mental State Examination (MMSE), or (5) had a score of 15 or higher on the Alcohol Use Disorders Identification Test, (6) had not evaluated the level of anxiety, and (7) had not completed the follow-up assessment of delirium. The researchers consecutively enrolled a sample of 372 individuals undergoing THA with a total of 325 for analysis (see this exemplar study Figure 1). Enrolling consecutive patients is a reasonably unbiased way of obtaining a sample because it does not allow anyone on the research team to pick and choose who is in the study. In this study, consecutive enrollment of patients does not present any obvious concerns about the sample being different from persons who have THA at other times.	p. 2

		Page
Measurement and Quality of Data	The researchers provide clear descriptions of the scales used to measure anxiety, delirium, and other risk factors of POD. References are provided for validity and reliability of the scales.	pp. 2–3
	The demographic data, lifestyle, clinical characteristics, and MMSE were recorded on admission by the trained research assistant with patient interview and chart review. They assessed the level of the anxiety in the afternoon of the day before surgery with the HADS-A. The general anesthesia was performed in all participants. The surgical procedures were provided by one surgical team to avoid the bias from surgical procedures. The surgeons and anesthesiologists were blinded to the information about grouping. The assessment of the delirium was performed on the first 7 days after surgery as well as the duration and the severity. In participants with the development of the delirium, the severity was assessed using the MDAS and the duration was measured by days.	
Data Analysis	Descriptive statistics were used to summarize data according to the allocation. Missing data from the cases not assessing anxiety and delirium were deleted from the analysis. Student's t-test for normally distributed data, the Mann-Whitney U test for ordinal data without a normal distribution, and $\chi2$ tests for proportion distributions to compare the anxiety group and non-anxiety group. p-value < 0.05 was considered statistically significant. Variables that achieved significance on univariate logistic regression analysis were entered into multivariate logistic regression analysis to estimate the risk of postoperative delirium.	pp. 3–4

(continues)

		Page
	The multiple logistic regression analysis was used to adjust for multiple risk factors and interactions. Odds ratio (OR) and 95% confidence interval (CI) were presented to evaluate risk factors.	
Ethics Review	Ethical approval for this study [2019-N(H)-100] was provided by the biomedicine ethics board of the University of Science and Technology of China (USTC), Hefei, China (Chairperson Professor Liu) on March 5, 2019. The study was registered at the Chinese Clinical Trial Registry (ChiCTR) with the number of ChiCTR1900026054. Note the IRB approval number and clinical trial number are provided. These numbers are often required by many journals for publication.	p. 2
Results (What)		
Sample	In a cohort study, the first table often profiles the two cohorts as a first step in identifying potential confounders. Accordingly, Table 1 provides a profile of the baseline characteristics of 325 adults allocated to anxiety or non-anxiety groups with specifics about variables the researchers think (based on research evidence) could have an influence on the occurrence of complications. First, note that the anxiety cohort comprised 30% of the sample and the non-anxiety cohort made up the rest (70%). Then, there are differences between the composition of the two groups, particularly in terms of demographic, lifestyle, and clinical characteristics. This raises a concern that perhaps these differences influenced the occurrence of complications and contributed to the differences found. At this point, the differences just send up a red flag and remind us to note whether the researchers deal with them during data analysis.	pp. 3–4
Findings	Primary Outcomes In the text, the researchers tell us that 25.3% of patients with anxiety (82/325) and 14.8% of patients with no clinical anxiety (48/325) had a higher incidence of POD.	pp. 3–6

		Page
	Thus, the absolute difference in POD of the two groups is 10.8% (25.3% minus 14.8%). Further, the *p*-value associated with this difference indicates that this is a real difference, not a chance difference ($p = 0.025$).	
	To provide additional clinical perspective on the risk of POD, the risk for patients with anxiety to develop POD was compared to the risk for patients with no clinical anxiety.	
	The results were reported using a statistic called odds ratio. The analysis had to be done with odds ratios rather than risk ratios because of the technical requirements of logistic regression, which analyzes several risk factors at once. First, let us consider the concept of odds, the concept of risk, and how odds compare to risk.	
	■ The odds ratio (OR) is a comparison of the odds of an event after exposure to a risk factor with the odds of that event in a control or reference situation. The OR is estimated as the odds of an event in the exposure group divided by the odds of that event in the control or reference group; the result is expressed as a ratio to denominator. The statistical significance of an OR is stated along with the OR and its 95% confidence intervals (CIs). If the 95% CI for the OR includes 1.00, the OR is not statistically significant.	
	■ The relative risk (RR) of an event is the likelihood of its occurrence after exposure to a risk variable as compared with the likelihood of its occurrence in a control or reference group. The RR is estimated as the absolute risk with the risk variable divided by the absolute risk in the control group. It is almost invariably expressed as a ratio to denominator 1 rather than as a percentage. RR values are accompanied by their 95% CIs. lies within the range of the confidence interval. Odds of a complication Odds	

(*continues*)

		Page
	of a complication are similar to risk of a complication but slightly different. A risk is the likelihood (i.e., probability) of something occurring in relation to the number of times it could have occurred. You roll a die (just one) and are hoping to roll a five. There is one chance in six that you will get a five; thus, the risk of a five is one in six, which is 0.17 when converted to a decimal (1/6 = 0.166) and rounded up. In contrast, odds are the chances of something occurring in relation to the chances of it not occurring; thus, the odds of rolling a five are one to five (1/5) or 0.20. The numerator is the same in both calculations, but the denominator is different. Like relative risk, an odds ratio is a ratio, specifically the odds of a particular outcome occurring in the exposed group (the numerator) relative to the odds of it occurring in the unexposed group (the denominator). For practical purposes, they can be interpreted similarly as they both are ratios representing the association between the frequency of an outcome occurring in two groups. An RR or OR of 1 means the two groups had the same risk or odds of experiencing the particular outcome. A value greater than 1 means the exposed group had a greater likelihood of the outcome than the baseline group and a value less than 1 means the exposed group had a lesser likelihood. Therefore, an RR or OR of 4.0 means that the exposed group had four times the risk of the unexposed group, i.e., were four times as likely to experience the outcomes as those in the unexposed group. An RR or OR of 0.75 means the exposed group had 0.75 times the risk of the outcome compared to those who had no exposure. Said differently, the exposed group had a 25% reduction in risk compared to those without the	

		Page
	exposure. Because of the different denominator, RR and OR of an outcome will not be identical. In the exemplar study the odds ratio is reported and not the RR because of the type of regression analysis which analyzes several risk factors at once. As a clinical reader, you are not expected to know when one or the other should be used. The researcher and the peer review team are responsible for getting this right. For practical purposes, RRs and ORs can be interpreted similarly as both are ratios representing the association between the frequency of an outcome occurring in two groups. Getting back to the primary outcomes and Table 2 in the report, we notice that the OR and 95% CI are only reported in the text and not in Table 2. This is probably to save space. However, the report OR 0.51, 95% CI 0.92–0.29, $p = 0.025$ indicates a significant difference between patients with anxiety and those with no clinical anxiety. There is statistically significance because the 95% CI for the OR did not include 1.0. Therefore, a THA patient or postoperative patient with anxiety is the primary risk factor that determined whether POD as a primary outcome occurred. This analysis in essence ruled out the other risk factors as confounders, leaving anxiety as the best explanation for why POD occurred at different rates in the anxiety and no clinical anxiety THA groups. Potential Confounders The researchers controlled for potential confounders in order to clarify the relationship between POA and POD. The potential confounding factors, such as the emergency surgery and the history of cognitive impairment, that might interfere with the results were strictly controlled in the study. Additionally, the alcohol and smoke use, education level, pain, and the surgery time, which might affect the	

		Page
	incidence of the POD, were recorded and showed no statistical differences. Running a multiple logistic regression analysis helped address the differences between anxiety and no clinical anxiety patients or other risk factors influencing POD.	
	Secondary Outcomes	
	In the text and Table 2, the researchers report "the duration and severity of the POD had no statistical differences between two groups ($p = 0.518$ and $p = 0.397$, respectively). However, the LOS were longer in the POD patients with anxiety than the POD patients without anxiety [7.8(3.0) vs. 6.4(1.6), $p = 0.025$]. No differences were found in the other variables between two groups."	
	Postoperative outcomes in all participants	
	In the text and Table 3, the researchers showed the postoperative variables in all participants of the study. "The LOS was significantly longer in the anxiety participants than those without clinical anxiety ($p = 0.038$), suggesting that the POA might prolong the recovery time from the surgery due to the longer length of stay. There were no statistical differences in the other variables between those two groups, including admitting to ICU, transfusion, surgery time, and other postoperative complications."	
	Delirium risk factors	
	The logistic regression model was performed to find the predictors of the POD. In the text and Table 4, the researchers report results of the multivariate logistic regression model. Age ($p = 0.012$), alcohol abuse ($p = 0.013$), history of stroke ($p = 0.031$), scores of the HADS-A ($p = 0.030$), and education level ($p = 0.034$) were considered to be the predictors of the POD. From a statistical perspective, statistically significant at the $p < 0.05$ level. This means that there is a 5% chance that a difference as large as the one found could have occurred just by chance—thus a difference is likely to	

		Page

exist in the larger population as well as in this sample. Note in Table 4 that the 95% confidence intervals are provided for each variable. Interpreting the CI, we would say we are 95% confident the interval (1.009–1.074) captured the true mean age (52.2). The CI provides a better sense of what might occur in the population than does the sample mean all by itself.

At this point, if you do not understand confidence intervals, you should go back to your statistical text because you are likely to encounter them when reading research reports and SRs. They are of practical, clinical value because they provide good estimates of the likely results that will be realized when applying the study's intervention in everyday practice. A specific confidence interval gives a range of plausible values for the parameter of interest.

Wrap-up of OR and RR

To sum up the OR and RR explanations, you don't have to know how to calculate ORs and RRs or even the technical difference between them, but you should know how to interpret their meanings. Hopefully, from the use of OR in this article and explanation of each in this profile and commentary you know how to do that. You may find that RRs and ORs have a commonsense meaning if you just remember that:

1. The key word to understanding ORs and RRs is the word relative.
2. You need to note which group is the baseline/unexposed group, i.e., the denominator.
3. An OR or RR with 1 in the confidence interval means that the two groups have the same frequency of having the outcome.
4. A value greater than 1 means that the numerator group has a greater likelihood of the outcome than the baseline group and a value less than 1 (and 1 is not in its confidence interval) means a lesser likelihood of the outcome.

(continues)

		Page
Discussion	Importantly, the researchers placed their findings in the context of other work that has been done on the subject and concluded that the findings of this study add to the list of studies showing that POA predicted the incidence of POD in patients undergoing THA.	p. 7

References

D'Andrea, E., Vinals, L., Patorno, E., Franklin, J. M., Bennett, D., Largent, J. A., Moga, D. C., Yuan, H., Wen, X., Zullo, A. R., Debray, T. P. A., & Sarri, G. (2021). How well can we assess the validity of non-randomised studies of medications? A systematic review of assessment tools. *BMJ Open, 11*(3), Article e043961. https://doi.org/10.1136/bmjopen-2020-043961

Simin, J., Liu, Q., Wang, X., Fall, K., Williams, C., Callens, S., Engstrand, L., & Brusselaers, N. (2021). Prediagnostic use of estrogen-only therapy is associated with improved colorectal cancer survival in menopausal women: A Swedish population-based cohort study. *Acta Oncologica, 60*(7), 881–887. https://doi.org/10.1080/0284186X.2021.1909747

Vafaei, H., Karimi, Z., Akbarzadeh-Jahromi, M., & Asadian, F. (2021). Association of placental chorangiosis with pregnancy complication and prenatal outcome: A case-control study. *BMC Pregnancy and Childbirth, 21*(1), Article 99. https://doi.org/10.1186/s12884-021-03576-0

Vaughn, V. M., Gandhi, T. N., Chopra, V., Petty, L. A., Giesler, D. L., Malani, A. N., Bernstein, S. J., Hsaiky, L. M., Pogue, J. M., Dumkow, L., Ratz, D., McLaughlin, E. S., & Flanders, S. A. (2021). Antibiotic overuse after hospital discharge: A multi-hospital cohort study. *Clinical Infectious Diseases, 73*(11), e4499–e4506. https://doi.org/10.1093/cid/ciaa1372

CHAPTER 9

Systematic Reviews

Once several or many studies have been conducted on a problem, clinicians or researchers will pull together the findings of these studies into a summary to see the big picture. This pulling together is called a **systematic literature review,** most often shortened to a systematic review. When done well, a systematic review helps clinicians and researchers identify what is known with certainty, what is tentatively known, and what the gaps in knowledge are about a problem. Not infrequently, systematic reviews serve as a link between individual studies and clinical decision making and between individual studies and clinical practice guidelines.

Sometimes a well-conducted systematic review calls into question a widely used clinical practice method. Other times it confirms the effectiveness of existing practice. In the following example you'll note that the studies are old, but they provide a good example of practice effectiveness confirmation.

A systematic review of studies examining the effectiveness of rapid response systems included 29 eligible studies. The results for adults were a reduction in cardiopulmonary arrests outside intensive care units and a reduction in hospital mortality outside of ICUs (Maharaj et al., 2015). The reduction in adult hospital mortality was in contrast to an earlier systematic review that found no reduction in this outcome (Chan et al., 2010).

Types of Systematic Reviews

A standard or consensus definition of a systematic review does not exist. To create a starting point for proposing an explicit and non-ambiguous systematic review definition, Krnic Martinic et al. (2019) conducted a systematic review and analyzed the definitions of a systematic review in healthcare literature as well as the elements of the definitions that are. The authors, proposed definition reads:

"A systematic review is a review that reports or includes the following:

1. Research question
2. Sources were searched with a reproducible search strategy (naming of databases, naming of search platforms/engines, search date and complete search strategy)
3. Inclusion and exclusion criteria
4. Selection (screening) methods

5. Critically appraises and reports the quality/risk of bias of the included studies
6. Information about data analysis and synthesis that allows the repro-ducibility of the results" (Krnic Martinic et al., 2019).

There are three ways of summarizing results across studies:

1. Systematic review with narrative synthesis
2. Systematic review with statistical synthesis
3. Systematic review with qualitative synthesis

Synthesis in this context is the combining of the results of multiple individual studies to produce conclusions that represent the body of results. Said differently, it is a new whole (group of conclusions) produced from the parts (results of individ-ual studies). Although the goal of all three methods of a systematic review is to use rigorous methods to produce integrated conclusions about what is known and not known about a problem, their methods of analysis and synthesis are different. The differences are necessary because the essential nature of clinical issues varies widely and therefore are studied using different study designs, which produce results in different forms.

- Systematic reviews with narrative synthesis analyze and summarize the find-ings of studies with various types of quantitative data. The adjective *narrative* refers to the fact that the analysis and synthesis are done using logical reasoning and text (in contrast to statistics).
- Systematic reviews with statistical synthesis referred to as a **meta-analysis**, are used to combine the results of experimental studies of treatments and in-terventions by statistically pooling data to produce an estimate of the direction and size of the treatment effect. The Preferred Reporting Items for Systematic Reviews and Meta-Analyses (PRISMA) provides evidence-based minimum sets of items for reporting systematic reviews (Page et al., 2021).
- Systematic reviews with qualitative synthesis aim to identify trends in the find-ings of qualitative studies so as to develop deeper and more complete under-standings of social, psychological, and experiential phenomenon. The enhancing transparency in reporting the synthesis of qualitative research (ENTREQ) pro-vides reporting guidelines for qualitative systematic reviews (Tong et al., 2012).

Although all three types of systematic reviews produce essential knowledge for practice, narrative synthesis in systematic reviews are also called state-of-the-science summaries; narrative reviews are more commonly found in clinical nursing jour-nals. Thus, narrative synthesis in systematic reviews will be the focus of this chapter and again later in the text. Examples of the other two types of systematic reviews SRs are posted on the student website.

Close and Distant Relatives of Narrative Synthesis in Systematic Reviews

You will find articles in the nursing literature called **scoping reviews or integrative research**. Scoping reviews address an exploratory research question by completing a knowledge synthesis to map key concepts, types of evidence, and research gaps. While scoping reviews may be conducted under the value and scope of systematic reviews, they differ in that authors do not have single or precise questions; they are most interested in identifying specific concepts in papers or studies and in mapping, reporting, or discussing these characteristics/concepts (Munn et al., 2018). Integrative research reviews are quite variable in that some self-identify as integrative research reviews but would qualify as systematic reviews with narrative synthesis. Integrative reviews summarize past empirical or theoretical literature to comprehensively understand a particular phenomenon or healthcare problem. Integrative reviews thus have the potential to build nursing science, informing research, practice, and policy initiatives. The integrative review method allows for the inclusion of diverse methodologies (i.e., experimental and non-experimental research) (Munn et al., 2018).

Scoping and integrative research reviews are more likely than narrative synthesis in systematic reviews to include both qualitative and quantitative studies and many integrative reviews incorporate conceptual and theoretical sources; this is not a negative, rather, it serves to integrate research and theoretical perspectives. Generally speaking, to qualify as a narrative synthesis in systematic reviews, an integrative research review report should explicitly and transparently describe the review methods used, appraise study quality, and summarize findings (Snyder, 2019).

Before heading into a description of how systematic reviews are produced, we want to point out that all three types of systematic reviews are different from literature reviews in several ways (see **Table 9-1**), including:

- Prescribed criteria regarding how a systematic review should be done have been established. Additionally, systematic review reports include detailed descriptions of each step in the production process. In contrast, no production process is prescribed for literature reviews; rather, they are done according to the reviewers' predilections. Moreover, there is no expectation that the production process is described. The lack of a prescribed process for literature reviews and the lack of detailed reporting about how they are done increase the likelihood that they are prone to bias.
- Systematic reviews incorporate only research reports. Literature reviews typically include a wide variety of articles, including essays, anecdotal accounts, and opinion.
- Systematic reviews are based on an exhaustive and diligent search for studies, whereas literature reviews can be, and often are, selective in what they report.
- Systematic reviews use a **quality filter** either to exclude poor-quality studies or to categorize the quality of studies included; literature reviews do not do this.

Table 9-1 Differences Between Systematic, Scoping, Integrative, and Literature Reviews

Feature	Systematic Review	Scoping Review	Integrative Review	Literature Review
Purpose	Thorough examination of a specific issue	Map the body of literature on key concepts	Summarize past empirical or theoretical literature	Highlights of an issue; varying degrees of thoroughness

(continues)

Table 9-1 Differences Between Systematic, Scoping, Integrative, and Literature Reviews *(continued)*

Feature	Systematic Review	Scoping Review	Integrative Review	Literature Review
Production Process	Standards exist and the process used is described in report	Standards exist and a modified PRISMA flow diagram is required	No standards and current methods of analysis, synthesis, and conclusion drawing remain poorly formulated	No standards; process not described
Search	As exhaustive as possible	Based on inclusion/exclusion criteria with necessary changes	Comprehensive but with a specific focus	Often limited
Inclusion	Original study reports, previous systematic reviews, information from large databases	May involve multiple structured searches rather than a single structured search	Purposive sampling of data which includes original studies and grey literature	Original study reports, theoretical literature, essays, opinion articles
Selection	Should use a quality appraisal filter	Based on inclusion/exclusion and is broader than systematic reviews. Quality filter not used.	Based on identified problem or question. Inclusion of empirical and theoretical reports and diverse study methodologies. Quality filter not used	Quality filter not used
Report	Inclusive of all qualifying studies	A logical diagram or table that aligns with the scope of the review. May include numerical summary and qualitative thematic analysis.	Qualitative/ narrative synthesis for qualitative and quantitative studies	Often selective based on purpose (cherry picking)

The Systematic Review Production Process

To judge whether a systematic review conclusion is a sound basis for care, you need to be aware of the standards for producing them. The steps taken to produce all three types of systematic reviews are as follows:

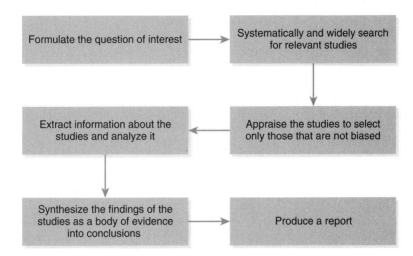

These steps are in accordance with the more detailed process standards set by internationally recognized organizations: Cochrane Collaboration (Higgins & Thomas, 2022); Eden et al. (2011); Joanna Briggs Institute (2014); Page et al., (2021). These standards have been outlined in detail to control error and bias. The early steps are similar in all systematic reviews, but data extraction, analysis, and synthesis are different for each type of systematic review.

Formulate the Topic and Assemble a Panel

Panels or individuals with expertise in the issue of interest conduct systematic reviews. The word *conduct* is used because doing a systematic review is demanding and rigorous. A panel has greater potential to conduct a systematic review that is free of error and bias than does an individual because the panel members act as checks and balances to each other's work and uncover unconscious bias.

Scope

Typically, a professional organization identifies the topic, issue, or problem its members think needs summarization. The **scope** of systematic reviews varies; sometimes the topic is broad; other times the issue is relatively narrow. A broad topic addresses several aspects of an issue, whereas a narrow topic focuses on one aspect.

For instance, a broad review about preventing falls in home-dwelling elders would have to include studies regarding the functional status of patients (e.g., balance and gait), the role of medications, orthostatic hypotension, environmental issues, and more. In contrast, a narrower review about environmental alterations to prevent falls in the home could focus on a smaller subset of studies having to do with floor surfaces, grab bars, lighting, steps, and so on. The broad and narrow scope is not a good–bad issue; the scope depends on what clinicians in the area of practice need to know and what has already been summarized. However, broader topics require more resources to conduct the review, are more difficult to summarize, and require more extended reports.

Types of Studies

Early on, the panel considers the types of studies they will include in the systematic review and how far back they will go in the search for studies and previous systematic reviews. Sometimes changing technology or patterns of care signify that it does not make sense to go back beyond a specific date.

Reviewers can decide to include studies using the full range of designs or just those with specific design characteristics. For instance, a research group interested in obtaining the best estimates of the effects of colchicine on major adverse cardiovascular events performed a systematic review and meta-analysis of randomized trials (Bytyci et al., 2021). In contrast, a research group interested in identifying and synthesizing frontline nurses' experiences and challenges when caring for patients with COVID-19 in hospitals used only qualitative studies (Thomas et al., 2021). The clinical issue of interest determined the difference in the types of studies included in the two reviews.

In the recent past, when conducting a systematic review about a clinical treatment or intervention, the interest was merely in treatment effectiveness, thus, only randomized studies, that is, experimental studies, were included. Increasingly, however, researchers are recognizing the need to go beyond summarizing studies about the treatment effect to address other issues related to the treatment such as problems patients have following a particular treatment regimen and how the treatment affects their daily lives. These are essential considerations when evaluating the evidence supporting a treatment. They shed light on its actual use. Real patient-world effectiveness of a treatment or intervention is most likely a combination of direct physiological or psychological effectiveness and patient response and use factors.

Studies about these real-world issues are conducted using qualitative and nonexperimental methods. Thus, increasingly, organizations producing systematic reviews are working on how qualitative and nonexperimental quantitative studies can be used to inform and add to the information obtained from randomized controlled studies (Cochrane Collaboration, 2015).

Early on, systematic review panels decide how they will handle studies of dubious or poor methodological quality. Some panels will include them but note their poor or modest quality, whereas others will eliminate them. Still, others will analyze the results of low-quality and high-quality studies together and then separately to determine if study quality affects the conclusions.

Search for Studies and Screen for Relevance

The search for studies begins when the topic and scope have been clearly specified. Most review panels include a health science librarian with expertise in locating research reports. The most common search starting place is the computerized **databases** of the published healthcare literature (CINAHL, MEDLINE, PsycINFO, and others). Reviewers typically search several healthcare databases using various search terms, combinations of search terms, and search options.

Usually, the panel's initial goal is to identify all potential studies on the issue; however, database indexing and retrieval may fail to identify some eligible studies, which can be a source of bias. Moreover, databases include only published studies, and some studies may have been done but not published. Thus, retrieval of eligible studies from databases is only a starting point. In an attempt to include findings from all relevant studies, panels often peruse reference lists, check research registries and conference presentations, contact colleagues, and even run searches using web search engines.

At this point, hundreds of citations may be under consideration. A careful reading of abstracts can reduce the number considerably by eliminating those that are not research reports or are not on topic. Then, all potentially relevant research reports are retrieved. Using a prespecified set of inclusion–exclusion criteria, two or more persons decide which studies are eligible for the systematic review. The PRISMA 2020 flow diagram for new systematic reviews is often required and is a great tool for mapping the flow of information through the different phases of a systematic review (Page et al., 2021). (See **Figure 9-1**.)

Appraise

All of the eligible studies should then be carefully appraised for quality; the goal of this appraisal is to eliminate studies that are biased or not credible because of the study methods. The number of studies that survive relevance screening and quality appraisal may be much smaller than the number initially identified during the search phase. It is not uncommon to have hundreds of citations identified by the search, but end up with 30, or even 8 studies, in the final review. The Grading of Recommendations Assessment, Development, and Evaluation (short GRADE) is one tool that can be used to grade the quality (or certainty) of evidence and the strength of recommendations (Schünemann et al., 2013).

Extract and Analyze

The panel will then sort the final body of research reports into stacks by key questions or subtopics, such as those using similar forms of the intervention or those evaluating a particular clinical outcome. For instance, a study measuring effectiveness in community-based palliative care programs looked separately and together at community-based, palliative care, advanced illness management, and advanced care and supportive care (Vernon et al., 2022).

Evidence tables are typically required for systematic reviews and are a great tool in taking evidence-based practice from the page into the clinical setting. Basic information about design, sample, variables studied, and results are carefully extracted from the report and entered into evidence tables. There are many different types of evidence or literature tables. However, the main thing is to determine the essential pieces that help draw out the comparisons and contrasts between the articles included in the review. The first few columns should include the basic info about the article (title, authors, and journal), publication year, and the purpose of the paper. Lists or coding may help identify differences, commonalities, and patterns across the studies. Different research questions, contexts, ways of measuring a variable, or timing of the outcome measurement are noted. Similarities and differences in findings are identified, and reasons for the variations are explored. (See **Table 9-2**.)

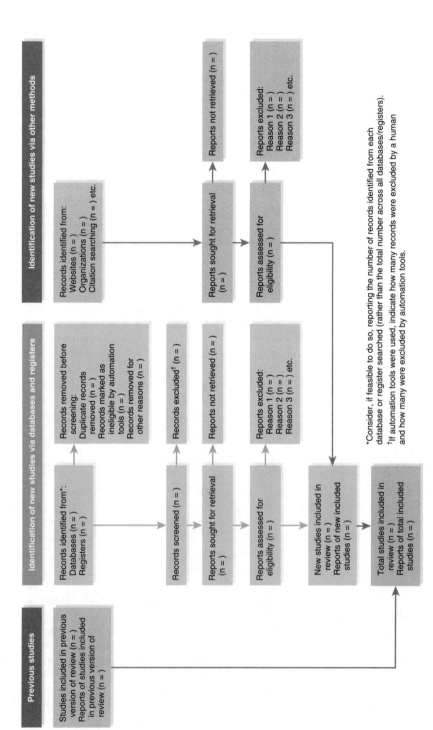

Figure 9-1 PRISMA 2020 Flow Diagram

Data from Page. M. J., Moher, D., Bossuyt, P. M., Boutron, I., Hoffmann, T. C., Mulrow, C. D., Shamseer, L., Tetzlaff, J. M., Akl, E. A., Brennan, S. E., Chou, R., Glanville, J., Grimshaw, J. M., Hróbjartsson, A., Lalu, M. M., Li, T., Loder, E. W., Mayo-Wilson, E., McDonald, S., . . . McKenzie, J. E. (2021). PRISMA 2020 explanation and elaboration: Updated guidance and exemplars for reporting systematic reviews. *BMJ, 372*, Article n160. https://doi.org/10.1136/bmj.n160. This article is published under a CC-BY Creative Common License https://creativecommons.org/licenses/by/4.0

Table 9-2 Example of a Narrative Synthesis in Systematic Reviews Evidence Table from Exemplar Study

Study	Methods	Setting	Participants	Interventions	Outcomes	Findings
Neunhoeffer et al.[38] 2015	Pre/post quasiexperimental study: convenience sample	Medical–surgical–cardiac PICU, University Children's Hospital, Tübingen, Germany	N = 337 165 = pre-implementation of protocol 172 = post-implementation of protocol Inclusion criteria: 0–18 years Exclusion criteria: Post-surgical patients, death, tracheostomy, or transfer to another hospital	Review of pain/sedation scores and opioid administration pre and post-implementation of a nurse-titrated sedation protocol to determine if it is effective in providing adequate sedation. Pre-implementation: Analgesia and sedation were managed by the order of the attending physician. While nurses could communicate their opinions and observations regarding the patient's sedation requirements, they were not authorized to change the sedation regimen without a physician's order. Standard therapy before and after implementation: 5–100 mcg/kg/hr with starting dose 30 mcg/kg/hr. Post-implementation: NCA using a nurse driven protocol for sedation and analgesia.	Measurement: Cumulative amount of opioid consumption calculated in standardized morphine equivalents and measured as mcg/kg/hr. Sedation was rated using the COMFORT-B tool with scores 6–30. Target score [12–18]. NISS was also used [1–3]. Score of 2 is an indicator of adequate sedation. IWS was measured by the SOS. Scores _ 4 indicative of withdrawal.	Authors' conclusion: The incidence of withdrawal symptoms in critically ill children decreased significantly with the use of a nurse-driven protocol. Reviewers' comments: Unsuccessful attempt to contact author to provide further information. Number of neonates in study unknown. With no data for this participant subset, unable to extrapolate results to a neonate population.

Table 9-2 Example of a Narrative Synthesis in Systematic Reviews Evidence Table from Exemplar Study   *(continued)*

Study	Methods	Setting	Participants	Interventions	Outcomes	Findings
Deeter et al.[34] 2011	Pre/post quasiexperimental study: convenience sample	PICU, Seattle Children's Hospital University of Washington, Seattle, USA	N = 319 153= pre-implementation of protocol 166 = post-implementation of protocol Inclusion criteria: 0–21 years Exclusion criteria: Diagnosis of seizures; acute or chronic neurologic dysfunction; extracorporeal life support; tracheostomy in place for any part of the ICU admission; infusion of a neuromuscular blocking agent; transfer from another ICU; or death during admission.	Intervention: Review of pain/sedation scores and opioid administration pre- and postimplementation of a nurse titrated sedation protocol to determine if it is effective in providing adequate sedation. Pre-implementation: Analgesia and sedation were managed by the order of the attending physician. Post-implementation: NCA using a nurse driven protocol for sedation and analgesia.	Measurement: Duration of opioid exposure in days.	Authors' conclusion: A nurse driven protocol can significantly reduce sedation and analgesic use. Reviewers' comments: Unsuccessful attempt to contact author to provide further information. Number of neonates in study unknown. With no data for this participant subset, unable to extrapolate results to a neonate population.

Reproduced from Muirhead, R., Kynoch, K., Peacock, A., & Lewis, P. A. (2021). Safety and effectiveness of parent- or nurse-controlled analgesia in neonates: A systematic review. *JBI Evidence Synthesis, 2021*), 3–36. https://doi.org/10.11124/JBIES-20-00385

Synthesize/Conclude

The goal of synthesis is to reach conclusions representing the findings of the individual studies as elements of a body of findings, which is different from looking at each one in isolation from the others. Combining findings from many studies in the form of integrated conclusions is referred to as *synthesis* because new knowledge claims are produced—claims that go beyond what any single study produced. The term *synthesis* makes the process of bringing research findings together sound exacting, which is not quite the reality. In the conduct of all three forms of systematic reviews, even when the reviewers are conscientious, interpretation is inherent in the process; assumptions, decisions about inclusion and exclusion, and faulty reasoning can affect the conclusions, and even produce misleading ones. However, these sources of bias can be minimized by following the recognized ways of conducting narrative synthesis in systematic reviews.

Synthesis involves integrating the findings considering differences, similarities, and relative methodological quality. In the case of narrative synthesis in systematic reviews, the integration is achieved using inductive reasoning to produce conclusions, which are new findings. In the case of systematic reviews with meta-analysis, the data from the original studies are extracted and pooled for the statistical analysis that evaluates the overall direction and size of the effect. Often, the statistical estimate of treatment **effect size** (point estimate and 95% confidence interval) for each study in the systematic review is shown in a graph that makes clear how many studies found a benefit, how many found no benefit, and how enormous the benefit or lack of it was. For those readers interested in understanding the results of a meta-analysis, several references are provided on the text website; alternatively, you can search online for "meta-analysis forest plots."

Report

Narrative synthesis in systematic reviews reports open by stating the issue they examine and why the reviewers think it is essential. You should note if the review focused on a specific population or setting and whether it is focused on one or several outcomes. For instance, a review about the effectiveness of relaxation techniques could focus just on the outcome of pain, or it could also include studies that examined relaxation techniques for anxiety, onset of panic attacks, or smoking cessation.

Next, the process that was used to search for study reports is described in detail, including databases searched, key terms used, and any inclusion or exclusion criteria used. The number of records identified, included, and excluded, and the reasons for exclusions should be indicated, often using a flow diagram such as that in Figure 9-1. The process used to extract information from the reports and the methods used to evaluate the quality of the studies should also be described.

Typically, tables display much-abbreviated profiles of the studies and their findings. Table 9-2 is part of the evidence table from this chapter's exemplar study (Muirhead et al., 2021). Note how this table provides a quick overview of the methods and the results of the studies.

In the text, consistent, conflicting, and equivocal findings, as well as gaps in the research base, are reported and bottom-line conclusions are set forth. Finally, the panel or authors indicate whether and how their conclusions square with any prior work that has been done on the topic, summarize the limitations of the body of research, and offer opinions regarding the clinical implications of the conclusions.

Use of a Narrative Synthesis in Systematic Reviews

Narrative synthesis in systematic reviews are published in clinical journals with increasing frequency, which is very helpful to clinician teams designing nursing protocols. Locating a well-conducted, recent narrative synthesis in systematic reviews saves a clinical project team all the work of identifying, retrieving, appraising, analyzing, and summarizing the research findings for the protocol they are designing.

At the same time, users of narrative synthesis in systematic reviews need to keep in mind that the conclusions are interpretations of findings. Two review groups examining the same research findings could arrive at different conclusions. From the search of studies to the appraisal of the quality of the individual studies and the conclusions, there are numerous points at which the opinion of two review groups could differ. One group may discount the findings of a study that another group thinks is important. One group may focus on one outcome, while another thinks another outcome is more important. Often the conclusions are similar or complementary, but sometimes they are contradictory.

Umbrella Systematic Reviews

Some issues have been the topic of several, even many, systematic reviews; thus, overviews of existing systematic reviews are appearing in the healthcare literature—often referred to as **umbrella reviews**. Many of these reviews address a broad scope of issues related to a topic of interest and present a comprehensive picture of the research evidence related to a particular question. Some umbrella reviews summarize existing research syntheses (Joanna Briggs Institute, 2014), whereas others produce new knowledge by combining information, patterns, and inconsistencies in the existing reviews into new conclusions (Conn & Coon Sells, 2014). The methods for conducting umbrella reviews are rigorous, however because they are aimed at busy clinicians, they often use a minimum of text to convey conclusions and tables to summarize the characteristics and findings of the individual systematic reviews they examine (Walsh et al., 2022). As an example, a systematic review of 55 existing systematic reviews aimed to inform future guidelines by exploring the impacts of maternal-focused interventions on infant feeding. The researchers concluded there is sufficient evidence to justify greater inclusion of mothers in more holistic packages of care for small and nutritionally at-risk infants aged <6 months (Von Salmuth et al., 2021).

Healthcare organizations around the world produce and index systematic reviews. In Chapter 12, you will learn how to search for them, and in Chapter 15, you will learn how to appraise the quality of narrative synthesis in systematic reviews.

Exemplar

Systematic Review Exemplar Article

Muirhead, R., Kynoch, K., Peacock, A., & Lewis, P. A. (2021). Safety and effectiveness of parent- or nurse-controlled analgesia in neonates: a systematic review. *JBI Evidence Synthesis, 20*(1), 3–36. https://doi.org/10.11124/JBIES-20-00385

Systematic Review Analysis and Application Table

		Page
Study Purpose (Why)		
Methods (How)		
Design	Search Strategy and Sample Guidelines for Reporting Quality Appraisal	
Data Analysis		
Results (What)		
Findings		
Discussion	Limitations	

Systematic Review Profile and Commentary on the Exemplar Article

Muirhead, R., Kynoch, K., Peacock, A., & Lewis, P. A. (2021). Safety and effectiveness of parent- or nurse-controlled analgesia in neonates: A systematic review. *JBI Evidence Synthesis, 20*(1), 3–36. https://doi.org/10.11124/JBIES-20-00385

		Page
Study Purpose (Why)	The authors are quite clear in the abstract and introduction sections regarding why they thought this systematic review needed to be done. The problem or gap is that increased opioid analgesia use to relieve neonate's pain is associated with numerous complications, such as iatrogenic withdrawal syndrome (IWS).	Abstract pp. 5–6
	One effective strategy for managing neonatal pain is with the use of parent- or nurse-controlled analgesia (P/NCA).	
	Research evidence indicates that the P/NCA is effective in lower opiod dosages, and decreased pain. However, no systematic review of P/NCA use in neonates has been completed. Therefore, the reviewers of this systematic review aimed to determine the safety and effectiveness of P/NCA on neonatal patient outcomes. They specifically list out the review's objectives and questions. See exemplar pp. 5–6	
Methods (How)		
Design	Search Strategy and Sample	pp. 6–11
	This systematic review has a detailed methodology that describes the search process and the selection process. The review methods used are in line with widely recognized recommendations, in accordance with the JBI methodology, and followed the steps set forth earlier in this chapter. The review included both experimental and quasi-experimental study designs. The reviewers list out inclusion criteria for participants, intervention, compactor, and outcomes. Of interest, the reviewers made modifications from the protocol to include several other studies to ensure inclusion of all studies that examined P/NCA in the neonatal population. This is not unusual for a systematic review to identify studies during the review and make modifications to include them.	

		Page
	Guidelines for Reporting	PRISMA Flow Chart
	This review reflects the stages outlined in the protocol. The search used the usual databases. The reviewers describe study inclusion in the text and per recommendations of PRISMA, a flow chart of the selection process is provided (p. 9). Supplementary to the flow chart, the reviewers provide a detailed list of ineligible studies with a reason for the exclusion in appendix II. Some of the reasons for exclusion were that the study did not include neonatal participants or the study used different study designs.	
	Quality Appraisal	GRADE p. 4
	Importantly, all studies included in the review were appraised in detail for methodological quality using GRADE standards (an internationally recognized grading system for quality of evidence) and JBI grading tools. Risk of bias across studies was assessed. The summary of findings on p. 4 presents the GRADE and then appraisal results of the 14 included studies are presented in **tables 1–4**, pp. 10–11. The reviewers included all studies regardless of methodological quality due to the paucity of neonatal data; however, they provide detailed explanations of the low-quality methodological issues. Ultimately the low quality of the studies led the authors to lack confidence in their findings and to be tentative in their conclusions.	**Tables 1–4**
Data Analysis	The reviewers provide sufficient information, critical reflection, and interpretation from each study findings within the text and within an evidence table located in appendix III. The study selection was performed independently by two reviewers, ensuring interrater agreement and these reviewers further read and extracted, recorded the studies in detail, enhancing integrity of the dataset. The reviewers provide a through and creditable analysis of the data.	pp. 8–18 Appendix III
Results (What)		
Findings	The reviewers grouped the results according to the primary outcomes of pain intensity, opioid consumption, occurrence of IWS, and adverse events. Within each of these groups the studies were compared; the details are provided in the tables and in the text. The reviewers summarize and point out patterns and	pp. 8–18

(continues)

		Page
	limitations across studies. For example, they point out that the study results indicate reduced neonatal pain with opioid administration and P/NCA managed pain in neonates, however, certainty is limited due to heterogeneity. Heterogeneity means that there is variability within the data, such as instruments or measurement tools, study design, or populations. The same reporting format was used for the other groups.	
Discussion	The reviewers then provide detailed, meaningful, and original discussion on pain intensity, opioid consumption, occurrence of IWS, and adverse events. The reviewers' interpretation of the main findings does not repeat the results.	pp. 18–21
	Strengths, weaknesses, and comparisons with literature answer this review's research question and whether the hypothesis was confirmed. For example, the certainty of the other study findings is reduced because of the small study sizes and varied opioid administration and dosages.	p. 21
	Several limitations are discussed. The reviewers mention that the level of evidence varied across studies. There was considerable heterogeneity of interventions and measurements for outcomes in all studies. Lastly, the use of different opioids and variability in conversion rates may have over- or underestimated the amount of opioid received. However, despite the limitations, each still provided or contributed to new knowledge.	
Conclusion	This systematic review provides an answer to the research question and significance of the findings. The reviewers conclude, that the results suggest P/NCA tailored and responsive analgesia may maintain effective pain control while reducing opioid administration and consumption.	pp. 21–22
	The reviewers then remind us of the limitations; however, the review still has implications and recommendations for further practice and research. For example the reviewers recognize future NICU studies are needed. These studies should include standard NICU training and services.	

References

Bytyci, I., Bajraktari, G., Penson, P. E., Henein, M. Y., & Banach, M. (2021). Efficacy and safety of colchicine in patients with coronary artery disease: A systematic review and meta-analysis of randomized controlled trials. *British Journal of Clinical Pharmacology, 88*(40), 1520–1528. https://doi.org/10.1111/bcp.15041

Chan, P. S., Jain, R., Nallmothu, B. K., Berg, R. A., & Sasson, C. (2010). Rapid response teams: A systematic review and meta-analysis. *Archives of Internal Medicine, 170*(1), 18–26. https://doi.org/10.1001/archinternmed.2009.424

Cochrane Collaboration. (2015). Cochrane Qualitative & Implementation Methods Group. http://methods.cochrane.org/qi/

Conn, V. S., & Coon Sells, T. G. (2014). WJNR welcomes umbrella reviews. *Western Journal of Nursing Research, 36*(2), 147–151. https://doi.org/10.1177/0193945913506968

Eden, J., Levit, L., Berg, A., & Morton, S. (Eds.). (2011). *Finding what works in health care: Standards for systematic reviews.* National Academies Press. https://doi.org/10.17226/13059

Higgins, J. P. T., & Thomas, J. (Eds.). (2022, February). *Cochrane handbook for systematic reviews of interventions* (Version 6.3.0). The Cochrane Collaboration. https://training.cochrane.org/handbook/current

Joanna Briggs Institute. (2014). *Reviewers' manual.* Author. https://nursing.lsuhsc.edu/JBI/docs/ReviewersManuals/ReviewersManual.pdf

Krnic Martinic, M., Pieper, D., Glatt, A., & Puljak, L. (2019). Definition of a systematic review used in overviews of systematic reviews, meta-epidemiological studies and textbooks. *BMC Medical Research Methodology, 19*(1), Article 203. https://doi.org/10.1186/s12874-019-0855-0

Maharaj, R., Raffaele, I., & Wendon, J. (2015). Rapid response systems: A systematic review and meta-analysis. *Critical Care (London, England), 19*(1), Article 254. https://doi.org/10.1186/s13054-015-0973-y

Muirhead, R., Kynoch, K., Peacock, A., & Lewis, P. A. (2021). Safety and effectiveness of parent- or nurse-controlled analgesia in neonates: A systematic review. *JBI Evidence Synthesis, 20*(1), 3–36. https://doi.org/10.11124/JBIES-20-00385

Page, M. J., Moher, D., Bossuyt, P. M., Boutron, I., Hoffmann, T. C., Mulrow, C. D., Shamseer, L., Tetzlaff, J. M., Akl, E. A., Brennan, S. E., Chou, R., Glanville, J., Grimshaw, J. M., Hróbjartsson, A., Lalu, M. M., Li, T., Loder, E. W., Mayo-Wilson, E., McDonald, S., . . . McKenzie, J. E. (2021). PRISMA 2020 explanation and elaboration: Updated guidance and exemplars for reporting systematic reviews. *BMJ, 372,* Article n160. https://doi.org/10.1136/bmj.n160

Munn, Z., Peters, M. D. J., Stern, C., Tufanaru, C., McArthur, A., & Aromataris, E. (2018). Systematic review or scoping review? Guidance for authors when choosing between a systematic or scoping review approach. *BMC Medical Research Methodology, 18*(1), Article 143. https://doi.org/10.1186/s12874-018-0611-x

Schünemann, H., Brożek, J., Guyatt, G., & Oxman, A. (Eds.). (2013). *GRADE handbook for grading quality of evidence and strength of recommendations.* The GRADE Working Group, 2013. https://gdt.gradepro.org/app/handbook/handbook.html

Snyder, H. (2019). Literature review as a research methodology: An overview and guidelines. *Journal of Business Research, 104,* 333–339. https://doi.org/10.1016/j.jbusres.2019.07.039

Tong, A., Flemming, K., McInnes, E., Oliver, S., & Craig, J. (2012). Enhancing transparency in reporting the synthesis of qualitative research: ENTREQ. *BMC Medical Research Methodology, 12*(1), Article 181. https://doi.org/10.1186/1471-2288-12-181

Thomas, N., Coleman, M., & Terry, D. (2021). Nurses' experience of caring for patients with delirium: Systematic review and qualitative evidence synthesis. *Nursing Reports (Pavia, Italy), 11*(1), 164–174. https://doi.org/10.3390/nursrep11010016

Vernon, E., Hughes, M. C., & Kowalczyk, M. (2022). Measuring effectiveness in community-based palliative care programs: A systematic review. *Social Science & Medicine, 296,* Article, 114731. https://doi.org/10.1016/j.socscimed.2022.114731

Von Salmuth, V., Brennan, E., Kerac, M., McGrath, M., Frison, S., & Lelijveld, N. (2021). Maternal-focused interventions to improve infant growth and nutritional status in low-middle income countries: A systematic review of reviews. *PloS One, 16*(8), e0256188. https://doi .org/10.1371/journal.pone.0256188

Walsh, J., Dwumfour, C., Cave, J., & Griffiths, F. (2022). Spontaneously generated online patient experience data—how and why is it being used in health research: An umbrella scoping review. *BMC Medical Research Methodology, 22*(1), 139. https://doi.org/10.1186/s12874-022-01610-z

CHAPTER 10

Evidence-Based Clinical Practice Guidelines

Position papers and care **guidelines** have been used by healthcare professionals for clinical conditions in their specialty for years without a standard for how these guidelines are developed. At times, recommendations were based on one or several studies combined with a good amount of expert opinion. However, over the last decade, the use of research evidence to support clinical guidelines has become a standard made possible by the vastly accessible research studies and systematic reviews about a variety of clinical topics.

Evidence-based clinical practice guidelines can be summarized as a set of recommendations for a specific clinical topic that are used to optimize patient care. These recommendations are informed by a systematic review of the evidence (Chapter 9) and consider the benefits and harms of other care options (Graham et al., 2011). Here's a short list of nursing-relevant evidence-based clinical practice guidelines, just to give you a sense of what is being produced:

- *Respectful Maternity Care Framework and Evidence-Based Clinical Practice Guideline* (Association of Women's Health, Obstetrics, and Neonatal Nurses, 2022).
- *Nurse Retention for Nurse Managers* (Tang & Hudson, 2019).
- *Pain Assessment for Older Persons in Nursing Home Care* (Sirsch et al., 2020).
- *Central Line–Associated Bloodstream Infection Prevention* (Conley, 2016).

Although evidence-based clinical practice guidelines are technically a translation of research evidence, in the real world, if they are well-produced, they are considered research evidence. So, when the term *research evidence* is used, it refers to recommendations of evidence-based clinical practice guidelines, conclusions of systematic reviews, and findings of original individual studies.

In this chapter, evidence-based clinical practice guidelines are used instead of evidence-based practice (EBP) to make clear that the guidelines being described are based on available research evidence complemented by expert opinion when necessary. Most guideline developers recognize expert opinion as evidence; however, it is considered a lower level because it is subjective.

Subjective evidence is much like the testimony of a reliable eyewitness of an event; better than no witness but not as strong as physical evidence. The credibility of expert opinion within evidence-based clinical practice guidelines is heightened as the opinions are that of the whole guideline development panel, not just one individual.

Forerunners to Care Protocols

Evidence-based clinical practice guidelines are generic in that they are not designed for a particular organization or agency; rather, they are offered as guidelines for care in a variety of settings. Although evidence-based clinical practice guidelines can be used by individual clinicians, they are often adapted by clinical project teams into care protocols specific to their setting, patients, and staff. These care protocols serve as standards of care in providing evidence-based guidance for care providers. Importantly, standardizing the processes of care based on research evidence has the potential to:

1. Increase the use of clinical actions that are effective.
2. Reduce the use of actions that are of minimal value or put patients at risk.
3. Reduce undesirable variation in care.
4. Reduce unnecessary waste in healthcare resources.

These kinds of process of care improvements have been found to improve patient safety, quality of care, and patient outcomes (Cassidy et al., 2021). Care protocols take many forms, including standardized care plans, care maps, decision algorithms, care bundles, standard order sets, clinical procedures, and clinical pathways. Increasingly, they are being incorporated into healthcare organizations' electronic decision support and communication systems.

Lest you be concerned that *standardized plan of care* sounds like a cookie-cutter care whereby every patient with a particular problem automatically gets the same care regardless of their unique characteristics and wishes, be assured that patient-centered care and standardized plans of care *are* compatible. This is done through the nurses' observations and response to patient needs, desires, and wishes while giving care in accordance with standardized plans. If the care recommended by the standardized plan is not acceptable to the patient or the patient is not responding well, it is acceptable for the nurse to collaborate with their clinical leader about how to proceed. It should also be said that most caregiving organizations expect professional caregivers to exert judgment and consider the individual patient's condition, preferences, life situation, and personal goals when planning and giving care. Standardized plans of care benefit most but not necessarily all patients.

Evidence-based clinical practice guidelines are an intermediate step on the rather long road from individual studies to evidence-based practice (see **Figure 10-1**). One of the biggest benefits to the use of an evidence-based clinical practice guideline for a project team developing a care protocol rather than systematic reviews is that evidence-based clinical practice guidelines save time. The group's expertise and translation of the research evidence to recommended care actions expedites the development of a plan for incorporating the recommendation or recommendations into the organization's care processes.

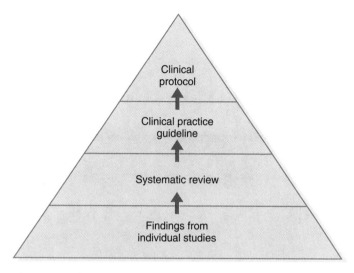

Figure 10-1 Knowledge Transformations

Patient-centered care and standardized plans of care are compatible.

Evidence-Based Clinical Practice Guidelines Production

As part of the evidence-based practice movement, quality standards for the production process of evidence-based clinical practice guidelines have been formulated and are widely agreed upon. Multidisciplinary groups and professional associations in many countries provide manuals regarding the production of clinical practice guidelines (Australian Government National Health and Medical Research Council, n.d.; Graham et al., 2011; Guidelines International Network, n.d.; Registered Nurses' Association of Ontario, n.d.; Scottish Intercollegiate Guidelines Network, n.d.). While there are some differences of opinions and emphasis within the content of evidence-based clinical practice guidelines, the process does not differ much if at all. The production process can be lengthy, should be rigorous, and must have integrity in each and every step. Knowing the production process for evidence-based clinical practice guidelines will help you to appraise guidelines in the future as the production process is an important criterion for judging whether a guideline is trustworthy. Appraising evidence is something we will address in Part 2 of this text.

Purposes

The organization or association commissioning the development of a guideline typically sets specific goals for the project. A clear purpose statement assures that the development panel proceeds in sync and on mission. Later, it conveys to potential users of the guideline what they can expect from it. The purpose statement may include a health condition that requires management or prevention, a patient

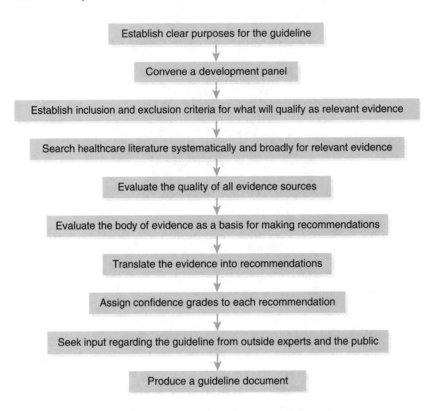

Establish clear purposes for the guideline

Convene a development panel

Establish inclusion and exclusion criteria for what will qualify as relevant evidence

Search healthcare literature systematically and broadly for relevant evidence

Evaluate the quality of all evidence sources

Evaluate the body of evidence as a basis for making recommendations

Translate the evidence into recommendations

Assign confidence grades to each recommendation

Seek input regarding the guideline from outside experts and the public

Produce a guideline document

population with a certain condition, or a specific care action or healthcare delivery process that requires procedural clarification.

Panel Composition and Expertise

Members are chosen to ensure that all affected healthcare stakeholders and the needed expertise are present at the table. That would include the following:

- Representation of all key professionals who will be influenced by the guideline.
- Clinical expertise in the various issues the guideline will address.
- Research expertise to help appraise study quality and interpret the study results.
- Evidence-based practice expertise to ensure sound transfer of knowledge from science to clinical recommendations.
- Information search and retrieval expertise to help locate research evidence.
- Group process expertise to facilitate the development process, group dynamics, and consensus decision making.
- For some guideline topics, a member of the public.

Inclusion and Exclusion Criteria

The inclusion-exclusion criteria are largely determined by the guideline's purpose, which may specify the target population, outcomes of interest, or setting characteristics. However, it may also include criteria regarding the types of study designs that will be included. It is not uncommon for guidelines to make recommendations regarding treatment or intervention effectiveness to include only randomized controlled studies. However, other study designs are included to recommend treatment issues other than effectiveness, such as helping patients adjust to the intervention.

Search for Evidence

The search for relevant evidence should be systematic and comprehensive. This undoubtedly requires the services provided by an information specialist or healthcare librarian skilled in searching health-related databases. Ideally, the search would identify systematic research reviews relevant to the guideline's issues. However, if relevant systematic reviews are not found or the ones found are not of acceptable quality or don't fully address the guideline's issues, reports of individual studies will have to be retrieved, and the development team will have to perform its own systematic reviews. These should be performed in accordance with recognized systematic review conduct standards as outlined in Chapter 9.

Evaluate Quality of All Evidence Sources

If working from existing systematic reviews, the panel should appraise their quality and use only those of acceptable quality. Appraising the quality of the individual studies in the systematic reviews is not required because good systematic reviews will already have done this. However, if the panel has to conduct its own systematic review, it would appraise the quality of the individual studies in producing it. Quality appraisal and eliminating poor quality evidence is critical in assuring trustworthy guidelines.

Evaluate the Body of Evidence

The panel then summarizes and evaluates the strength of *the body of evidence* on each problem about which it is considering making a recommendation. In so doing, the members should consider a wide range of characteristics of the body of evidence, which are listed in **Box 10-1** (Berkman et al., 2015; GRADE, n.d.). In the guideline document, the panel conveys its appraisal of the strength of the body of evidence by a combination of evidence tables, textual summarization of the evidence, or using an evidence-grading system that takes into account several characteristics of the body of evidence. It is challenging to capture all the characteristics listed in Box 10-1 with a simple grading system, so the grading systems in use either focus on several characteristics of the body of evidence or use grades that convey the quality and strength of the evidence in general terms. The strength-of-evidence rating systems in **Box 10-2** and **Box 10-3**, grade evidence related to interventions; note that they are quite different.

While the issue of whether the studies comprising the evidence were done using "the best design type" is important, it is just one aspect of the strength of the evidence. Until recently, evidence pyramids ranking evidence relied almost exclusively on the design of the studies. In these pyramids, which were designed mainly for evidence about interventions and treatments, a systematic review of randomized controlled trials, that is, experimental studies were ranked at the highest level followed by one or a few randomized controlled trials of good quality; nonexperimental and observational studies were ranked at a lower level. Now, evidence grading

Box 10-1 **Strength of a Body of Evidence**

To evaluate the strength of a body of evidence, the panel takes into consideration:

- Whether the studies done were of the best design type for the issue being considered.
- The methodological quality of the systematic reviews and/or the individual studies.
- The number of studies and/or systematic reviews.
- The consistency of the findings across studies.
- Whether enough patients were studied to confer confidence in the findings.
- If the estimated benefit of an intervention in the population is clinically significant.
- Whether population/s studied in the body of evidence are the same as the target population for the guideline.
- Whether the studies directly addressed important health outcomes.

Box 10-2 **Rating Scheme for Strength of Evidence**

Appraisal of Guidelines for Research and Evaluation (AGREE) II

The AGREE II is a critical appraisal tool that is used to measure the methodological rigour of the clinical practice guideline development. The instrument consists of 23 items organized within six domains, and two global rating items for an overall assessment. Each domain captures a specific aspect of guideline development quality.

Steps for Using Appraisal Tool:

The instrument guides users through six distinct domains. Each domain includes items that are scaled from 1–7, "strongly disagree" to "strongly agree". A quality score is calculated for each of the domains, with an overall score calculated by summing all the domains. The six domains are:

1. Scope and purpose: The overall aim of the guideline
2. Stakeholder involvement: The role and expectations of stakeholders
3. Rigour of development: The gathering and summarizing of the evidence
4. Clarity of presentation: The technical guidance
5. Applicability: The barriers and facilitators to implementation
6. Editorial independence: The identification of potential biases

Data from Brouwers, M. C., Kho, M. E., Browman, G. P., Burgers, J. S., Cluzeau, F., Feder, G., Fervers, B., Graham, I. D., Grimshaw, J., Hanna, S. E., Littlejohns, P., Makarski, J., Zitzelsberger, L., for the AGREE Next Steps Consortium. (2010). AGREE II: Advancing guideline development, reporting and evaluation in healthcare. *Canadian Medical Association Journal, 182*(18), E839-E842. https://doi .org/10.1503/cmaj.090449

Box 10-3 **Strength of a Body of Evidence Scale**

High

We are very confident that the estimate of effect lies close to the true effect for this outcome. The body of evidence has few or no deficiencies. We believe that the findings are stable, i.e., another study would not change the conclusions.

Moderate

We are moderately confident that the estimate of effect lies close to the true effect for this outcome. The body of evidence has some deficiencies. We believe that the findings are likely to be stable, but some doubt remains.

Low

We have limited confidence that the estimate of effect lies close to the true effect for this outcome. The body of evidence has major or numerous deficiencies (or both). We believe that additional evidence is needed before concluding either that the findings are stable or that the estimate of effect is close to the true effect.

Insufficient

We are unable to estimate an effect, or we have no confidence in the estimate of the effect for this outcome. The body of evidence has unacceptable deficiencies which preclude reaching a firm conclusion. If no evidence is available, it will be noted as "no evidence."

Reproduced from Agency for Healthcare Research and Quality. (2022, June 22). *Evidence-based practice center systematic review protocol: Project title: Radiation therapy for bone metastases.* Evidence-Based Practice Center (EPC) Reports. Author. https://effectivehealthcare.ahrq.gov/sites/default/files/product/pdf/rt-bone-metatases-final-protocol.pdf

systems, even those for interventions and treatments, take more than the design of the studies into consideration.

In addition, randomized controlled trials are not the best design for every guideline issue. In recognition of this fact, the Joanna Briggs Institute uses a levels-of-evidence approach that is composed of different levels of evidence ranking systems for: (1) intervention effectiveness; (2) diagnosis; (3) prognosis; (4) economic evaluations; and (5) meaning of human experience, interaction, and culture. The highest form of evidence is different for each of the five issues (Joanna Briggs Institute, 2014).

To summarize how the panel conveys the overall strength of the evidence about an issue: panels developing guideline documents should in some way grade the overall strength of evidence about each issue or question. If the evidence about an issue is moderate or high quality, the panel will usually recommend it.

Translate Evidence into Recommendations

To some extent, the detail of how the panel moves from evidence to a recommendation is a bit of a black box, typically described as "informal consensus." Understandably, many of the conversations required involve a tangle of evidence that lacks the consistency of populations studied, methods used, and results obtained, particularly certainty about the magnitude of benefit. Some developers are better at conveying what the panel discussed and took into account when making this translation. In the interests of transparency, the Institute of Medicine standards (Graham et al., 2011) require that development panels describe how decisions were made regarding whether or not to include a recommendation, how differences of opinion were resolved, and the part played by values, theory, and clinical experience.

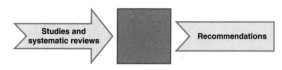

Assign a Certainty Level to Each Recommendation

Most guideline developers indicate the level of certainty they have in each recommendation. "When CPG developers are confident that the beneficial effects of a recommendation outweigh the harms, a strong recommendation can be made" (Graham et al., 2011, p. 113). The strength of the evidence supporting a recommendation is certainly a major consideration in determining how confident the panel is in a recommendation. However, other factors are also considered so that they can have certainty that the recommendation will produce desired patient outcomes without undue risk of harm and that the recommendations are feasible to use in practice (GRADE n.d.; Joanna Briggs Institute, 2014; U.S. Preventive Services Task Force, 2018; Dearholt & Dang, 2022). Some of the factors that enter into assigning a level of certainty to a recommendation are listed in **Box 10-4** and **Box 10-5**.

Box 10-4 **Certainty Considerations**

Issues considered in assigning a level of certainty to a recommendation:

- The strength or quality of the supporting evidence.
- Whether the populations and subpopulations to whom the recommendation would apply are clear.
- The size of the benefit likely to be achieved by the recommendation, i.e., it is clinically significant.
- The balance of benefits to risk of harm.
- Whether patients value the outcomes likely to be achieved.
- The cost and feasibility of implementing the recommendation.

Box 10-5 **Levels of Certainty Regarding Net Benefit**

Level of Certainty*	Description
High	The available evidence usually includes consistent results from well-designed, well-conducted studies in representative primary care populations. These studies assess the effects of the preventive service on health outcomes. This conclusion is therefore unlikely to be strongly affected by the results of future studies.
Moderate	The available evidence is sufficient to determine the effects of the preventive service on health outcomes, but confidence in the estimate is constrained by such factors as: The number, size, or quality of individual studies. Inconsistency of findings across individual studies. Limited generalizability of findings to routine primary care practice. Lack of coherence in the chain of evidence. As more information becomes available, the magnitude or direction of the observed effect could change, and this change may be large enough to alter the conclusion.

Level of Certainty*	Description
Low	The available evidence is insufficient to assess effects on health outcomes. Evidence is insufficient because of: The limited number or size of studies. Important flaws in study design or methods. Inconsistency of findings across individual studies. Gaps in the chain of evidence. Findings not generalizable to routine primary care practice. Lack of information on important health outcomes. More information may allow estimation of effects on health outcomes.

*The USPSTF defines certainty as "likelihood that the USPSTF assessment of the net benefit of a preventive service is correct." The net benefit is defined as benefit minus harm of the preventive service as implemented in a general, primary care population. The USPSTF assigns a certainty level based on the nature of the overall evidence available to assess the net benefit of a preventive service.
Reproduced from U.S. Preventive Services Task Force. (2018, October). *Grade definitions*. https://www.uspreventiveservicestaskforce.org/uspstf/about-uspstf/methods-and-processes/grade-definitions

Box 10-6 **Joanna Briggs Institute Grades of Recommendation**

Grade A	A "strong" recommendation for a certain health management strategy where (1) it is clear that desirable effects outweigh undesirable effects of the strategy; (2) where there is evidence of adequate quality supporting its use; (3) there is a benefit or no impact on resource use; and (4) values, preferences, and the patient experience have been taken into account.
Grade B	A "weak" recommendation for a certain health management strategy where (1) desirable effects appear to outweigh undesirable effects of the strategy, although this is not as clear; (2) where there is evidence supporting its use, although this may not be of high quality; (3) there is a benefit, no impact, or minimal impact on resource use; and (4) values, preferences, and the patient experience may or may not have been taken into account.

Reproduced from Joanna Briggs Institute Levels of Evidence and Grades of Recommendation Working Party. (2013, October). *JBI grades of recommendation*. https://jbi.global/sites/default/files/2019-05/JBI-grades-of-recommendation_2014.pdf

Some guideline developers use just two grades for their confidence in the recommendation (**Box 10-6**), while others use several levels. The recommendation grading system shown in **Box 10-7** is used by the U.S. Preventive Services Task Force (USPSTF), who assign one of five letter grades (A, B, C, D, or I) (2012). It considers the strength (amount of evidence) and compares benefit and harm.

Box 10-7 The U.S. Preventive Services Task Force (USPSTF) Grade Meaning and Suggestions for Practice

Grade	Definition	Suggestions for Practice
A	The USPSTF recommends the service. There is high certainty that the net benefit is substantial.	Offer or provide this service.
B	The USPSTF recommends the service. There is high certainty that the net benefit is moderate or there is moderate certainty that the net benefit is moderate to substantial.	Offer or provide this service.
C	The USPSTF recommends selectively offering or providing this service to individual patients based on professional judgment and patient preferences. There is at least moderate certainty that the net benefit is small.	Offer or provide this service for selected patients depending on individual circumstances.
D	The USPSTF recommends against the service. There is moderate or high certainty that the service has no net benefit or that the harms outweigh the benefits.	Discourage the use of this service.
I Statement	The USPSTF concludes that the current evidence is insufficient to assess the balance of benefits and harms of the service. Evidence is lacking, of poor quality, or conflicting, and the balance of benefits and harms cannot be determined.	Read the clinical considerations section of USPSTF Recommendation Statement. If the service is offered, patients should understand the uncertainty about the balance of benefits and harms.

Reproduced from U.S. Preventive Services Task Force. (2018, October). *Grade definitions*. https://www.uspreventiveservicestaskforce .org/uspstf/about-uspstf/methods-and-processes/grade-definitions

Ideally, guideline producers provide both a strength-of-evidence grade and certainty, or confidence, grade for each recommendation. However, other developers provide only a recommendation grade that considers the strength of the supporting evidence.

Input

Once the guideline document is in near-final form, the input should be sought from outside experts and the public. This review can identify a lack of clarity, omission of key issues, and questions about the feasibility of implementation. Some guideline developers put their guidelines through a field test; this helps determine whether the recommendations are implementable and what the barriers to implementation might be.

Ideas from outside reviews and field testing can lead to modification of the guideline document or adding suggestions that will help users put the recommendations in place.

Guideline Formats

Many guidelines are long. There are several reasons for this, including the following:

1. The broad nature of a guideline's purpose.
2. The inclusion in the guideline of details about the research evidence.
3. Inclusion of a description of the guideline production process.
4. Recommendations for practice, education, and organizations.

Although there is no standardized format for evidence based practice guidelines, the one that follows is typical:

1. Title.
2. Producing agency (date) and panel members.
3. Table of contents.
4. Copyright statement.
5. Background context.
6. Purpose and scope.
7. Practice recommendations.
8. Levels of evidence.
9. Definitions.
10. Discussion of evidence.
11. Evidence tables.
12. Production process.
13. Plans for updating.
14. Implementation strategies.
15. References.

To make guidelines more usable for clinicians, several of the elements just listed are often not included in the main document; rather, they are available in associated documents, often via online links. Even more convenient, evidence-based clinical practice guideline producers issue quick-reference guides separate from the full version of the guidelines. Quick-reference guides typically list the recommendations and indicate each recommendation's evidence grade or certainty level. The Joanna Briggs Institute produces two- to six-page best practice sheets, which are designed for clinicians; some are free to nonsubscribers (http://www.joannabriggslibrary.org/index.php/JBIBPTR). The Registered Nurses' Association of Ontario (n.d.) makes abbreviated versions of its guidelines available via its BPG app (http://rnao.ca/bpg/pda/app).

Because organizations and associations worldwide are producing evidence-based clinical practice guidelines, it is becoming more common for several guidelines to exist on the same topic. In response to this, several organizations have begun to produce syntheses of several guidelines. These syntheses lay out areas of agreement and difference and compare the recommendations. One of these syntheses, about the prevention of pressure ulcers, is available on the National Guideline Clearinghouse website (Agency for Healthcare Research and Quality, n.d.).

Comorbidity

Attention has been given to the reality that most guidelines address a single condition, whereas real-world patients often have several conditions (Harrison et al.,

2021). Few guidelines consider that many patients have several conditions (comorbidity) that could limit the applicability of a particular guideline to their care. An attempt to apply several guidelines to the care of a person with several conditions could result in the clinician being confronted by conflicting recommendations (Graham et al., 2011). Ultimately, addressing this dilemma will require changes in how research is conducted, how guidelines are developed, and the ability of the healthcare systems to support patient-centered care.

Guideline Producers

If you are interested in guidelines on a specific topic, five starting points for guidelines relevant to nursing would be:

- The Registered Nurses' Association of Ontario: http://rnao.ca/bpg
- The United States Preventive Services Task Force: https://www.uspreventive servicestaskforce.org/uspstf/
- The National Guidelines Clearinghouse: https://www.ahrq.gov/gam/index .html
- The University of Iowa College of Nursing Evidence-Based Practice Guidelines for Geriatric Care: https://nursing.uiowa.edu/news/9/18/2018
- The website of the professional association for your area of clinical interest; typically under the Practice tab

Exemplar

Evidence-Based Clinical Practice Guidelines Exemplar

Davidson, K., Barry, M. J., Mangione, C. M., Cabana, M., Caughey, A. B., Davis, E. M., Donahue, K. E., Doubeni, C. A., Epling, J. W., Kubik, M., Li, L., Ogedegbe, G., Pbert, L., Silverstein, M., Stevermer, J., Tseng, C.-W., & Wong, J. B. (2022). Screening for atrial fibrillation: US Preventive Services Task Force recommendation statement. *JAMA*, *327*(4), 360–367. https://doi.org/10.1001/jama.2021.23732

WWW

Evidence-Based Clinical Practice Guidelines Analysis and Application Table

		Page
Guideline Purpose (Why)		

		Page
Methods (How)		
Recommendations and Evidence (What)		

Evidence-Based Clinical Practice Guidelines Profile and Commentary

Davidson, K. W., Barry, M. J., Mangione, C. M., Cabana, M., Caughey, A. B., Davis, E. M., Donahue, K. E., Doubeni, C. A., Epling, J. W., Kubik, M., Li, L., Ogedegbe, G., Pbert, L., Silverstein, M., Stevermer, J., Tseng, C.-W., & Wong, J. B. (2022). Screening for atrial fibrillation: US Preventive Services Task Force recommendation statement. *JAMA, 327*(4), 360–367. https://doi.org/10.1001/jama.2021.23732

		Page
Guideline Purpose (Why)	This clinical guideline, issued by the U.S. Preventive Services Task Force (USPSTF), addresses three specific questions that are not explicitly stated in the Final Recommendation Statement reprinted but can easily be inferred from the objective statement, recommendations, and supporting evidence section. They are: 1. What are the benefits and harms of screening for AF in older adults? 2. What is the accuracy of screening tests, the effectiveness of screening tests to detect previously undiagnosed AF compared with usual care? 3. What are the benefits and harms of anticoagulant therapy for the treatment of screen-detected AF in older adults?	Abstract p. 361 pp. 363–365

(continues)

		Page
Methods (How)	The USPSTF's methods for producing a clinical guideline are available from a link on its home page: http://www.uspreventiveservicestaskforce .org/Page/Name/recommendations	pp. 360–362
	An 84-page USPSTF procedural manual describes the methods used to ensure that its recommendations are scientifically sound, reproducible, and well documented. Its production process is consistent with the ideal process set forth earlier in this chapter.	
	In the Supporting Evidence section, there is a statement that the USPSTF commissioned a systematic review to address the questions of interest. Having the SR in the guideline or as a supplemental document for reference is important for clinicians to see the evidence on which the recommendations are based. Supplemental content is linked on p. 360, right-side column. The Summary of Evidence section (particularly the evidence tables) of that report details the evidence for each supplement. Some clinicians will be interested in the details of the evidence whereas others will trust that the USPSTF followed its guideline production standards and accept the more general information about the evidence that is included in this Final Recommendation Statement document. The bottom line is: An extensive and rigorous systematic review was conducted and used as the evidence for the recommendations made.	
Recommendations and Evidence (What)	The Summary of Recommendation is displayed in the table right away on the first page. Note this brief summary details the population, the USPSTF's conclusion, and then provides an "I" for recommendation. Refer to your text and USPSTF's site for grade definitions.	pp. 360–363
	U.S. Preventive Services Task Force. (July, 2012). *Grade definitions*. Retrieved from https:// www.uspreventiveservicestaskforce.org/ uspstf/about-uspstf/methods-and-processes/ grade-definitions	
	You are directed to see the Practice Considerations section for additional information regarding the I statement.	

		Page
	Importantly, in the USPSTF Assessment of Magnitude of Net Benefit and Clinical Considerations section and Table of Summary of USPSTF Rationale, we learn that screening for AF in asymptomatic adults is lacking the evidence for harms and benefits. The table presents the rationale and assessment for the 3 question rationales with an eFigure in the Supplement for information on the recommendation grade used by USPSTF. Also, for more details on the methods the USPSTF uses to determine the net benefit, you are referred to the USPSTF Procedure Manual listed on the reference page.	
	Note that within the Table of Summary of USPSTF Rationale each of the 3 rationales have 2 assessments with only 2 of the 6 having adequate evidence to make a recommendation. Four of the 6 assessments have inadequate evidence to make a recommendation. Then the recommendation and how to implement the recommendation are explained in the Figure Clinician Summary: Screening for Atrial Fibrillation. This figure is also where you can find the link to read the full recommendation statement where more details on the rationale of the recommendation, including benefits and harms; supporting evidence (includes evidence table); and recommendations of others. It is a good idea to take a look at a full report to also see the design and complete methods used.	
	The guideline document conveys the patient population under consideration and each rationale in further detail under the practice considerations section. Then a definition for clinical AF is provided followed by considerations for screening tests. The screening tests were found to not have sufficient evidence; however, they outline several technologies proposed from the current evidence. They conclude that continuous or intermittent screening is more likely to detect AF; however, it is also more likely to detect short duration and paroxysmal AF.	
	Note, this conclusion is clearly stated in the Detection, Assessment part of the Table of Summary of USPSTF. Also, in the systematic review you can find the studies supporting this statement. For example, one study, of note, the trials listed both had good sample	

		Page
	sizes; however, the authors point out that the mean age for these trials ranged from 72–80 years.	
	The treatment and intervention section had two inadequate pieces of evidence; therefore, the reviewers speak to current treatment strategies. Importantly, they point out that the stroke risk instruments were not developed for screen-detected AF. The instruments were developed for patients with diagnosed AF.	
	You can refer to the systematic review and read that he USPSTF reports no trials found that report on anticoagulant benefits.	
	Then further read that and convey from these studies, due to either the trials not having screening or low sensitivity, the benefits of screening in detected populations is uncertain.	
	Lastly, the third harms section is addressed in the Suggestions for Practice Regarding the I Statement. In this section, the authors recognize the potential for preventable burden and potential for harm. They highlight that there is an increased risk of stroke for patients with AF not receiving anticoagulant therapy. Then, they point out that there is insufficient evidence to make a recommendation against or for AF screening. They, the USPSTF, then go into details on the risks and benefits for subclinical AF screening. Particularly, they highlight that some screening strategies might detect shorter duration or lower burden subclinical AF; however, these strategies are not completely clear. Also, they point out that is not completely clear which duration of subclinical AF would benefit from anticoagulant therapy.	
	For harms, the USPSTF reviewers point out that there is no associated harm using a wearable rhythm monitoring device.	
	However, of note, they also note that misdiagnosis could result from screening misinterpretation.	
	Then, you can note that anticoagulant therapy has a risk for bleeding. Together, the true-false positive results of ECG detection and some of the treatments have the potential for harm. For these reasons, based on benefits and harm, they could not conclude a recommendation whether AF screening should be or should not be completed in adults 50 or older without a diagnosis or symptoms of AF and without a history of transient ischemic attack or stroke.	

References

Agency for Healthcare Research and Quality. (n.d.). *Guidelines and Measures.* http://www.guideline.gov/syntheses/synthesis.aspx?id=47794

AGREE Next Steps Consortium (2017). *The AGREE II Instrument* [Electronic version]. http://www.agreetrust.org

Association of Women's Health, Obstetrics, and Neonatal Nurses. (2022). Respectful maternity care framework and evidence-based clinical practice guideline. *Journal of Obstetric, Gynecologic, and Neonatal Nursing, 51*(2), e3–e54. https://doi.org/10.1016/j.jogn.2022.01.001

Australian Government National Health and Medical Research Council. (n.d.). *Guideline development process.* https://www.nhmrc.gov.au/how-nhmrc-develops-public-health-guidelines

Berkman, N. D., Lohr, K. N., Ansari, M. T., Balk, E. M., Kane, R., McDonagh, M., Morton, S. C., Viswanathan, M., Bass, E. B., Butler, M., Gartlehner, G., Hartling, L., McPheeters, M., Morgan, L. C., Reston, J., Sista, P., Whitlock, E., & Chang, S. (2015). Grading the strength of a body of evidence when assessing health care interventions: An EPC update. *Journal of Clinical Epidemiology, 68*(11), 1312–1324. https://doi.org/10.1016/j.jclinepi.2014.11.023

Cassidy, C. E., Harrison, M. B., Godfrey, C., Nincic, V., Khan, P. A., Oakley, P., Ross-White, A., Grantmyre, H., & Graham, I. D. (2021). Use and effects of implementation strategies for practice guidelines in nursing: a systematic review. *Implementation Science: IS, 16*(1), 1–102. https://doi.org/10.1186/s13012-021-01165-5

Conley S. B. (2016). Central line-associated bloodstream infection prevention: Standardizing practice focused on evidence-based guidelines. *Clinical Journal of Oncology Nursing, 20*(1), 23–26. https://doi.org/10.1188/16.CJON.23-26

Dang, D., Dearholt, S., Bissett, K., Ascenzi, J., & Whalen, M. (2022). *Johns Hopkins evidence-based practice for nurses and healthcare professionals: Model and guidelines* (4th ed.) Sigma Theta Tau International.

Grading of Recommendations Assessment, Development and Evaluation Working Group. (n.d.). *The GRADE approach.* https://www.gradeworkinggroup.org/

Graham, R., Mancher, M., Wolman, D. M., Greenfield, S., & Steinberg, E. (Eds.). 2011. *Clinical practice guidelines we can trust.* National Academies Press. https://www.ncbi.nlm.nih.gov/books/NBK209539

Guidelines International Network. (n.d). *International Guidelines Library & Registry.* http://www.g-i-n.net/

Harrison, C., Fortin, M., van den Akker, M., Mair, F., Calderon-Larranaga, A., Boland, F., Wallace, E., Jani, B., & Smith, S. (2021). Comorbidity versus multimorbidity: Why it matters. *Journal of Multimorbidity and Comorbidity, 11*, Article 2633556521993993. https://doi.org/10.1177/2633556521993993

Joanna Briggs Institute. (2014). *New JBI levels of evidence.* https://jbi.global/sites/default/files/2019-05/JBI-Levels-of-evidence_2014_0.pdf

Registered Nurses' Association of Ontario. (n.d.). *Best practice guidelines.* https://rnao.ca/bpg

Sirsch, E., Lukas, A., Drebenstedt, C., Gnass, I., Laekeman, M., Kopke, K., Fischer, T., & Guideline workgroup (Schmerzassessment bei älteren Menschen in der vollstationären Altenhilfe, AWMF Registry 145-001) (2020). Pain Assessment for Older Persons in Nursing Home Care: An Evidence-Based Practice Guideline. *Journal of the American Medical Directors Association, 21*(2), 149–163. https://doi.org/10.1016/j.jamda.2019.08.002

Scottish Intercollegiate Guidelines Network. (n.d.). *Improving patient care through evidence-based guidelines.* https://www.sign.ac.uk/

Tang, J. H., & Hudson, P. (2019). Evidence-based practice guideline: Nurse retention for nurse managers. *Journal of gerontological nursing, 45*(11), 11–19. https://doi.org/10.3928/00989134-20191011-03

U.S. Preventive Services Task Force. (October 2018). *Grade definitions.* https://www.uspreventiveservicestaskforce.org/uspstf/about-uspstf/methods-and-processes/grade-definitions

Evidence-Based Practice

In Part 1, you acquired foundational knowledge about the different kinds of research studies that are used to study nursing phenomena, the features each type of research study offers, basic knowledge about how systematic reviews are completed, how evidence-based clinical practice guidelines are produced, and we hope, an appreciation overall for the incredible diversity of evidence available! Figure P2-1 graphically portrays the ground covered in the first part of the text. This knowledge is essential for using research evidence in your own nursing practice and for participating in evidence-based practice (EBP) projects in your work setting.

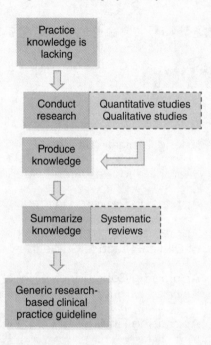

Implementing Research Knowledge

Research knowledge is not enough; you also need to be able to find research evidence, appraise it, and strategically use it in practice. That is what this second part of the text addresses. In Part 1, the focus was on the types of research evidence; as we move into Part 2, we'll pivot and consider "how do you use the evidence to make a change in practice?" If you are someone who likes to look ahead, you'll notice that the order of Chapters 14, 15, and 16 begins with the appraisal of evidence-based clinical practice guidelines (EbCPGs), then systematic reviews, then original, individual studies. This is the reverse of how you learned about them in Part 1 of the text. The reason for the reversal is that EbCPGs and systematic reviews are more reliable and ready for translation into practice, whereas the order in Part 1 was based on the natural learning order. To learn the appraisal process, we use the Johns Hopkins Nursing Evidence-Based Practice Model and Guidelines as an example of the many evidence-based practice models that exist in healthcare ([Johns Hopkins model] resources available @ https://www.hopkinsmedicine.org/evidence-based-practice /ijhn_2017_ebp.html). We've chosen this model due to the ease of use of their materials and their application to clinical scenarios. In Chapter 17, the lens is opened up, and you will learn how caregiving organizations use research evidence in combination with other types of evidence using the Johns Hopkins model and then in Chapter 18, we offer suggestions on how you personally can get involved (there are lots of different ways!)

In Chapter 19, the individual nurse's use of research evidence is described. The steps individual nurses use to incorporate research evidence into clinical decision-making for individual patients and to refine their own methods of practice are similar to those used by organizations, albeit performed with less rigor (Engle et al., 2021). Not all writers differentiate between evidence-based practice as an organizational activity and the individual's use of research evidence, but we think a distinction is important. A distinction between the two ways of using research evidence retains high standards for translating research evidence into clinical protocols while recognizing the value of individual nurses seeking better information when organizational protocols are lacking or are not applicable to a particular patient situation. The distinction also recognizes EBP as an organizational activity and **point-of-care design** as the individual professional nurse's responsibility. Maximally effective nursing care for patients requires translation of research into practice at both levels.

The Johns Hopkins Nursing Evidence-Based Practice Model

The Johns Hopkins model shown in Figure P2-2 depicts the major steps in achieving effective evidence-based practice in a healthcare organization. Importantly, each step should be thoughtfully and strategically carried out to ensure that the organizational protocol produced is truly evidence-based and that the implementation of the protocol has the desired effect on provider behavior and on patient outcomes. To achieve this level of translation of research evidence into practice, EBP projects are conducted by units, service lines, or agency teams composed of members with clinical, managerial, and EBP knowledge.

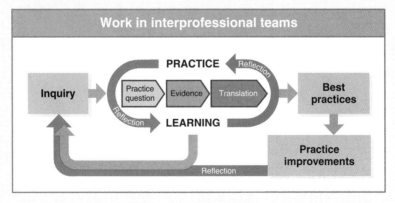

Reproduced from Dang, D., Dearholt, S., Bissett, K., Ascenzi, J., & Whalen, M. (2022). *Johns Hopkins evidence-based practice for nurses and healthcare professionals: Model and guidelines* (4th ed.). Sigma Theta Tau International.

The Johns Hopkins model is similar to other models that are used as working frameworks for the implementation of evidence-based practice programs in healthcare organizations. The Johns Hopkins model serves as a map for this part of the text.

References

Engle, R. L., Mohr, D. C., Holmes, S. K., Seibert, M. N., Afable, M., Leyson, J., & Meterko, M. (2021). Evidence-based practice and patient-centered care: Doing both well. *Health Care Management Review, 46*(3), 174–184. https://doi.org/10.1097/HMR.0000000000000254

Dang, D., Dearholt, S., Bissett, K., Ascenzi, J., & Whalen, M. (2022). *Johns Hopkins evidence-based practice for nurses and healthcare professionals: Model and guidelines* (4th ed.). Sigma Theta Tau International.

CHAPTER 11

Asking Clinical Questions

Evidenced-based nursing, simply put, means using evidence to guide daily nursing practice. Evidence-based practice (EBP) extends far beyond the clinical realm, from the classroom, where students learn how to be a nurse, to the boardroom, where nursing leadership makes decisions about the systems in which they work. For our text, we focus on clinical nursing, but the process outlined can be used regardless of what setting you find yourself in. Additionally, we've opted to use the Johns Hopkins Nursing Evidence-Based Practice Model (["Johns Hopkins model"]; Dang et al., 2022) as a framework or guide to the process, primarily because of the focus on nursing. The Johns Hopkins model is but one of many models that are useful in EBP; what model you use is of less consequence than having one to begin with.

The starting point for any team embarking on an evidence-based project is to understand what the issue or need is and then formulate a question in a way that will guide the search for research evidence and keep the project on target. In the Johns Hopkins model, this initial phase is called the inquiry phase (**Figure 11-1**).

Inquiry

Information pointing to an issue or need can come from various places in the system and prompt an inquiry to find more effective approaches. These inquiries occur within the PET process, or the "Practice – Evidence – Translation" process (Dang et al., 2022). Inquiries can be prompted by any number of sources including but not limited to staff members, quality management monitoring, risk management, financial reports, infection control monitoring, care coordinators, and patients. The prompts can also come from outside the system in the form of new standards of care from a professional association, regulatory agency, or accrediting organization.

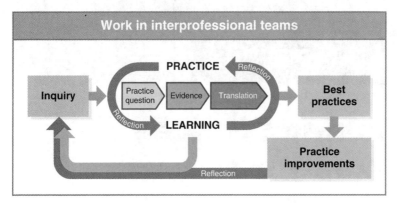

Figure 11-1 Inquiry phase

Reproduced from Dang, D., Dearholt, S., Bissett, K., Ascenzi, J., & Whalen, M. (2022). *Johns Hopkins evidence-based practice for nurses and healthcare professionals: Model and guidelines* (4th ed.). Sigma Theta Tau International.

Clinical Practice

Nurses and other care providers must be thoughtful, using critical thinking and clinical reasoning while giving care. Understanding why you are doing what you are doing and staying curious and committed to always seeking opportunities to do things better is key to optimizing quality care. What does this look like in practice? Have you ever asked yourself a question like:

- Should I recommend vitamin D supplements to my elderly patients?
- Should we be using bladder scans to determine urinary residual on all patients who have had an indwelling/Foley catheter removed?
- What nonpharmacologic measures can we use to prevent and treat muscle spasms in persons who have had cervical fusion surgery?
- Is acetaminophen or ibuprofen more effective and safer in treating fever in young children?
- What factors determine whether middle-aged men working in an industrial plant follow recommendations regarding how to avoid back injury?
- How do we create an environment for parents of premature infants that empowers them to be an active part of their child's activities of daily living?

If so, you are practicing that spirit of inquiry, or step one in the fluid Johns Hopkins model and even more exciting is what you can answer in part by examining the knowledge produced by research.

Quality Data

All healthcare systems collect a great deal of information to prove to third-party payers, accrediting agencies, and the public that the care given results in the patients achieving their desired outcomes. For example, a hospital might track the following information about people who have a discharge diagnosis of ischemic stroke:

- Readmission within 30 days
- Global disability status at discharge
- Discharge destination

- Special after-hospital services required
- Adverse events rates
- Complication rates

The system may also receive information from an accrediting agency, third-party payer, or a voluntary quality monitoring coalition about care and outcomes at other similar organizations. To be more specific: If a hospital's poststroke patients who were discharged on an anticoagulant medication had more emergency care visits for bleeding than similar patients discharged from other similar hospitals, the clinical staff would be obliged to reevaluate their teaching and discharge protocols for patients taking anticoagulants. If a current protocol was found not to represent current evidence-based standards of care, an EBP project to design a new protocol might be initiated. Thus, quality monitoring data, whether internal or shared, may shed light on a deficiency in care and serve as a prompt for an EBP project. Quality monitoring and its relationship to EBP is discussed more extensively in Chapter 17.

Professional Standards

When national professional associations issue evidence-based guidelines, systems are obligated to take notice and decide if they should change the way they are giving care. Similarly, when licensing and accrediting agencies, such as the Centers for Medicare and Medicaid Services (CMS) or the Joint Commission set new standards of care, systems have to decide how they will meet them which initiates a search for research evidence to help develop a new protocol. For example, in response to the recent COVID-19 pandemic, The Joint Commission began to score its new Standard IC.02.04.02 related to COVID-19 vaccination for healthcare staff, along with the applicable Medicare conditions of participation/conditions for coverage. This was in response to the Centers for Medicare and Medicaid Services (CMS) final rule "Omnibus COVID-19 Health Care Staff Vaccination" published in the *Federal Register* in November of 2021. This rule affected the Ambulatory Surgical Centers, Critical Access Hospitals, Hospitals, Home Care, Home Infusion Therapy, and Hospice Joint Commission programs. At a less formal level, a staff nurse might see an article or a research report in a clinical journal about a caring approach that seems promising. Or they may learn about a new guideline in a session at a conference or workshop. After thinking about the matter, they may conclude that this aspect of care as it is being done in their setting is of questionable effectiveness. Taking the concern and idea to a nurse leader, clinical nurse specialist, or case manager might lead to a search for research evidence about an alternative approach to care.

Questions Not Answerable by Research Evidence

Before looking at how to formulate a focused question for an evidence-based project, it might be helpful to address the kinds of questions that cannot be answered by research evidence.

One question that often cannot be answered with research evidence involves very new technology. If studies are available about new technology, they may have been conducted by the manufacturer and therefore should be appraised carefully for bias. An example would be if scientists could produce an external device that senses seizures just minutes before they occur; the early users of such a device would most likely have very little research evidence to go on.

The second question for which research evidence may not be available is the application of an existing intervention to a new population. There may be considerable evidence regarding the intervention in the population for which it was developed but none in the population with whom the system is considering using it. For instance, a digital device that monitors whether children use their asthma inhaler correctly may have been tested with children and found effective but may have yet to be tested in children with different abilities. Another example is when a body of research about the use of an intervention may have been conducted mainly with middle-class women, but there is little to no research about the use of the intervention with low inner-city women. In these situations, the research available is informative, but clinical protocols for the new population cannot be truly based on the available evidence.

The third type of question that cannot be definitively answered with research evidence is a question about the care of an individual patient who does not want a standardized intervention. The ethical principle is that each competent patient has the right to determine what happens to their person and body, and this principle must be respected regardless of what research evidence shows. Questions about what care should be given to an individual must be decided by the patient and their care providers. Research evidence can provide useful information to consider in the discussion, but ultimately the decision is the patient's or that of their designated healthcare proxy.

In light of the ethical principle just described, research evidence is also of limited use in questions having to do with values or deciding what is a moral or ethical course of action. The question, "Should we treat pneumonia in nursing home residents older than 90 years of age who have severe cognitive deficits?" is a moral question. Research may shed some light on the question by providing data regarding the percentage of this population that has an uncomplicated recovery and return to their former functional status when treated with antibiotics. However, research cannot answer the question. In fact, the question cannot be answered in general. It must be answered on a case-by-case basis because the answer depends on how cognitively compromised the person was before the onset of pneumonia, whether intubation is a likely possibility, and what the patient's end-of-life wishes were when last expressed—again, the ethical principle of self-determination. These ethical reminders are necessary to ensure that research evidence is used for the purposes it inherently serves and not as a means of controlling individual lives.

Forming a Useful Project Question

To keep the project on target and to avoid spending a lot of time searching for and sifting through a large number of citations, it helps to formulate a focused project question. One of the previously listed questions asked about creating an environment for parents of premature infants that empowers them to be an active part of their child's activities of daily living. This is a legitimate question, but it is vague and requires more focus. Let's assume that as a part of the process of determining the layout of a new NICU (Neonatal Intensive Care Unit), the NICU practice council decides to consider the research on this issue.

The council might use an approach that many healthcare providers have found useful in focusing their evidence-based clinical projects. This format is referred to by the mnemonic PICOT (Sackett et al., 2000; Stillwell, 2010). The PICOT format helps clinicians zero in on specific elements of a question that are of interest.

- **P** Patient population
- **I** Intervention/Issue
- **C** Comparison intervention
- **O** Outcomes
- **T** Timing

Generally, when using PICOT, the patient population can be characterized by attributes such as age, illness experience (e.g., shortness of breath), disease, or risk, to name a few. The intervention of interest can be specified by naming a clinical intervention, a particular approach, or a group of interventions (e.g., school-based programs regarding weight loss). For some questions, the *I* could stand for an issue rather than an intervention; this would be the case if the question was about mobility obstacles associated with foot drop. A comparison of the intervention to another intervention or to usual care may be of interest; alternatively, the effectiveness of just one intervention may be what is under consideration. Patient outcomes are almost always of interest, particularly outcomes that are important to patients, such as improved functional ability or fewer episodes of hypoglycemia. The timing, in terms of clinical status, duration, and frequency of treatment or length of follow-up, may be relevant. More recently, the addition of an "**S**" was added to the PICOT mnemonic (Samson & Schoelles, 2012).

- **P** Patient population
- **I** Intervention/Issue
- **C** Comparison intervention
- **O** Outcomes
- **T** Timing
- **S** Setting

This was done because specifying the setting of care can often help focus the question and reduce the number of citations retrieved that are not relevant. For instance, empowering parents within the home setting is significantly different than in the acute care setting.

Getting back to the issue of empowering parents within the NICU setting, a hospital practice council could develop a project question specific to NICU patients using **PICOTS** as follows:

For parents anticipating an extended length of stay in the NICU setting (P and S), does having private patient rooms (I) increase parental involvement in activities of daily living (O) over the course of the infant's stay (T) compared to shared rooms?

If you were to state this question specifying the outcome as "empowerment," you may not find many studies about it. So, it is possible to get too specific; sometimes some trial and error is required to get the question just right. Another example: Nurses on an obstetrical unit are concerned about the discomfort and distress newborns experience during and immediately after having blood drawn. To look into the intervention options, they formulated the following question:

> **What nonpharmacologic measures should nurses use (I) to reduce pain, discomfort, and agitation (Os) with full-term newborn infants (P) before, during, and after venipuncture and insertion of intravenous lines (T)?**

The intervention (nonpharmacologic measures) in this question is somewhat open-ended—and that's okay as it could identify measures of which the nurses were unaware. Alternatively, they may just be interested in comparing two methods, in which the question might be:

> **Is oral sucrose pacifier or swaddling more effective (I and C) in controlling pain (O) during and after venipuncture (T) in full-term newborns (P)?**

Note that the population specified in both questions is newborns, so the team looking into this issue would not retrieve or review guidelines, systematic reviews, and studies done on premature infants or infants older than 28 days.

Although not every clinical question about an intervention will have every PICOTS element, it is useful to at least consider each one. Generally, PICOTS works best for questions about intervention effectiveness. Questions regarding patients' experiences, the meaning of illness, relationships among clinical variables, and risk require modification of the PICOTS format. Nonintervention questions typically seek background evidence useful in developing assessment guides, teaching protocols, plans of care, or even whole programs. The *I* then represents *Issue* or *Issues,* instead of *Intervention.*

Let's consider another example; a project team at a stateside military hospital is opening a department to treat soldiers with traumatic brain injury. The team could formulate their question in several ways:

> 1. **In soldiers returning from combat with traumatic brain injury (P), what stateside rehabilitation setting characteristics (Issue and S) promote partner support and renewal of family relationships (Os)?**
> 2. **What issues and problems reconnecting with partner and families (Issue) are experienced by soldiers returning from combat with traumatic brain injury (P) to rehab units stateside (S)?**

The first question targets what the project team wants to know but research about it may not be available. The second question should access studies about the reuniting experiences of these returning soldiers to help the team comprehensively and deeply understand the soldiers' experiences and then develop setting-specific facilities and services that address them.

Sometimes project teams seeking evidence about background issues find it better to have two closely related questions rather than cramming the issues of interest into one question. For instance, a project team developing a support program for men with urinary incontinence might look at qualitative and descriptive studies about the experience of urinary incontinence and self-management strategies these men find helpful. The project questions could be:

1. **What experiences and self-management issues (I) do men with urinary incontinence (P) find stressful or difficult to manage (Os)?**
2. **What self-management actions and strategies help (Issue) these men (P) adjust to and cope with urinary incontinence (Os)?**

Together, these questions could result in retrieval of research evidence that would be useful in developing a clinical program that is patient centered and evidence based. Both questions have population, issue, and outcome elements but no comparison or time element.

What about a project group that seeks to develop a care protocol to support chronically ill mothers of young children; the questions guiding the project would be:

1. **When mothers of young children develop a chronic illness that affects physical functioning (P), how is their ability to mother their children affected (O)?**
2. **When mothers of young children become chronically ill (P), how do they and their partners (or immediate family) adjust to the situation (O)?**

Bottom line, make the project question as focused as possible by using the PICOTS format. If it turns out to be too specific (i.e., you cannot find any studies about it), you can either broaden one of the elements or drop it altogether. Doing so may open it up just enough that relevant evidence can be identified. If a project team has difficulty focusing its question, it is sometimes helpful to have several members spend a half hour muddling around in a database looking at various abstracts and articles about the issue. This muddling may help formulate a more focused question and help identify the terminology that will result in a productive search for evidence. After the team has a focused question that is consistent with the agency's commitments and resources, the next step is to search for research evidence related to that question. We'll address this in Chapter 12.

References

Dang, D., Dearholt, S., Bissett, K., Ascenzi, J., & Whalen, M. (2022). *Johns Hopkins evidence-based practice for nurses and healthcare professionals: Model and guidelines* (4th ed.). Sigma Theta Tau International.

Sackett, D. L., Straus, S. E., Richardson, W. S., Rosenberg, W., & Haynes, R. B. (2000). *Evidence-based medicine: How to practice and teach EBM* (2nd ed.). Churchill Livingstone.

Samson D., & Schoelles K. M. (2012, June). Developing the topic and structuring systematic reviews of medical tests: Utility of PICOTS, analytic frameworks, decision trees, and other frameworks. In S. M. Chang, D. B. Matchar, G. W. Smetana, & C. A. Umscheid (Eds.), *Methods guide for medical test reviews*. Agency for Healthcare Research and Quality. https://www.ncbi.nlm.nih.gov/books/NBK98241/pdf/Bookshelf_NBK98241.pdf

Stillwell, S. (2010). Asking the clinical question: A key step in evidence-based practice. *American Journal of Nursing, 110*(3), 58–61.

CHAPTER 12

Searching for Research Evidence

Searching for research evidence falls within the *evidence* step of the **Johns Hopkins model** P-E-T process. While we could spend a great deal of time talking about how to search the evidence, we've opted instead to provide some starting points so that you can learn by doing. So, where to start? The answer depends on the topic, how much time you have to devote to the search, and whether you are doing it as an individual or as part of a group. The search strategy that you use will also depend on the type of evidence you are looking for. This is driven by the practice question you are seeking to answer. You already know what types of evidence exist from Part 1; these include:

- Peer-reviewed and published research studies
    - Quantitative
    - Qualitative
    - Correlational
    - Experimental
    - Cohort
    - Systematic Reviews
    - Evidence-Based Clinical Practice Guidelines
- Community standards
- Opinions of internal and external experts
- Organizational financial data
- Position statements from professional organizations
- Patient and staff surveys and satisfaction data
- Quality improvement data
- Regulatory, safety, or risk-management data

It's important to state here that searching from the point of care on a handheld device will be different from an extensive search for an evidence-based project.

This chapter describes what is available from a health center or academic library. Point-of-care searching on handhelds will be addressed in Chapter 19.

Health Science Databases

First the basics: a database is a collection of a specified type of data that is organized for storage, accessibility, and retrieval. The specific type of data of interest to evidence-based nursing is bibliographic information about journal articles (and other resources) in the health sciences. Three of the most widely used databases by nurses are described below.

PubMed/MEDLINE

The most accessible database listing healthcare-related publications is PubMed. It is the online version of MEDLINE and is available at http://www.ncbi.nlm.nih.gov /pubmed/. Even simple searches using keywords are aided by pop-up suggestions. A PubMed search produces a list of relevant article citations, often with abstracts and sometimes with links for accessing the article (see the screenshot that follows).

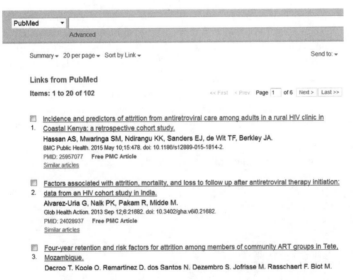

Reproduced from PubMed, National Center for Biotechnology Information, U.S. National Library of Medicine.

The PubMed search engine is quite powerful and has numerous features to help you get to the topic and evidence type of interest. Filters are available to help narrow your search by date, journal type, or language—to name just a few. Using the filter *Article type, Customize* you can limit your search to the evidence type you desire.

As with all the health science databases, it takes a bit of trial and error and practice to become proficient at using PubMed, but for those who rely on the Internet for their searching, the time would be well spent. To get you up to speed, the site provides a quick-start guide and tutorials.

For readers who have access to a health science library, you can access MEDLINE via the library's subscription. Most libraries have subscriptions to many journals, and often you can download the article right from the search engine the library uses. If a library doesn't have a subscription to a particular journal, the library can usually obtain the article you are interested in via other means.

Cumulative Index to Nursing and Allied Health Literature

The Cumulative Index to Nursing and Allied Health Literature, better known as CINAHL, is an index of articles in nursing and allied health journals and other resources that are not included in MEDLINE. However, there is considerable overlap between the two databases. CINAHL is available only by subscription, but all academic healthcare libraries and many hospital libraries have a subscription for students, their staff, and in many cases, members of the public. Many articles are available in full text. Like PubMed, you can do a simple search using keywords and combine them with *AND* or *OR*. You can then limit your search by article type, date of publication, or the age of the population of interest—just to name a few of the limits possible. Again, tutorials are provided, and most librarians will assist you in learning to navigate it.

PsycINFO

This database is centered on the interdisciplinary literature in psychology and the behavioral and social sciences. Many health science libraries subscribe to it, and it is searchable in many of the same ways as CINAHL. A fact sheet about it is available at http://www.apa.org/pubs/databases/psycinfo/psycinfo-printable-fact-sheet.pdf.

Nonprofit, International Organizations

If you are specifically looking for EbCPGs and systematic reviews, you'll find that quite a few independent international organizations produce or maintain databases of EbCPGs and systematic reviews. The following is a sampling of these organizations. These organizations are also mentioned in Chapter 10.

Registered Nurses Association of Ontario

This organization produces high-quality guidelines on a wide variety of topics. It uses an explicit and transparent production process. It has published and updated over 50 best practice guidelines, quite a few of which are available in languages other than English. Its guidelines are available free at its website, http://rnao.ca/bpg. It also offers condensed guidelines for mobile devices and implementation tool kits.

National Guideline Clearinghouse

The National Guideline Clearinghouse maintains an indexed database of clinical practice guidelines produced by a wide variety of organizations. The guidelines, which must meet inclusion criteria, are presented in a standardized format. Its index can be searched by disease/condition, by treatment/intervention, or by the health service sector (e.g., profession, geographic area, or by the organization producing the guideline). National Guideline Clearinghouse guidelines are available for free at http://www.guideline.gov/index.aspx.

U.S. National Preventive Services Task Force

This agency systematically reviews the evidence of effectiveness and develops recommendations for clinical preventive services. It offers an app to search for USPSTF recommendations by specific patient characteristics, including age, gender, and selected behavioral risk factors. Its website is http://epss.ahrq.gov/PDA/index.jsp.

Joanna Briggs Institute

The Joanna Briggs Institute is an international organization based in Australia with collaborating centers in over 40 countries. Its undertakings in the areas of developing and supporting the synthesis, transfer, and utilization of evidence is quite broad. Still, it does maintain a database of systematic reviews and implementation reports it and its international collaborating centers have produced. Most Joanna Briggs Institute resources are available only by subscription through a library; check to see if the library you use has a subscription. The Joanna Briggs Institute website is at http://joannabriggs.org/.

Cochrane Collaboration

Also an international organization, the Cochrane Collaboration promotes evidence-informed health decision making by producing high-quality systematic reviews. The Cochrane Database of Systematic Reviews includes reviews produced by the Cochrane Collaboration and its partner groups. SRs are free for all readers immediately after publication. You can search their open-access guidelines at http://www.cochrane.org/search/site.

Professional Specialty Organizations

Many professional specialty organizations produce and make available EbCPGs and SRs. Some organizations publish their guidelines in a book that can be purchased; others make them free to members, and others make their guidelines free online. The rigor of guideline development across the many producers varies. The list is long, but here are a few that make guidelines available for free online:

- American College of Physicians: https://www.acponline.org/
- Best Evidence Topics (BETs) Emergency Medicine: http://bestbets.org/home/bets-introduction.php
- Emergency Nurses Association: https://www.ena.org/
- HIV Medicine Association: http://www.hivma.org/hiv_guidelines/
- Oncology Nursing Association: https://www.ons.org/practice-resources/pep

Wrap-Up

Obviously, many sources are available. The secret to locating research evidence relevant to your project is to become proficient in using at least one database and then identifying a few other sources that issue or index EbCPGs and systematic reviews related to your clinical topic. We encourage you to poke around a bit to see what is applicable to your interests and to seek your librarian for consultation; they are wonderfully knowledgeable and eager to assist!

CHAPTER 13

Appraising Research Evidence

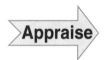

Assuming that your database searches resulted in the retrieval of at least one clinical practice guideline, systematic review, or report of an individual study, the next step is to appraise its quality to determine if you can have confidence in it. In this chapter, we'll provide an overview of how to appraise your evidence using the **Johns Hopkins model tools** and then determine whether it is worthy of including in your recommendations. You can access the **Johns Hopkins model tools** both in a writable format and in an electronic format at https://www.ijhn-education.org /node/18409#overlay-context=node/18409 after consenting to the noted legal conditions on the webpage.

Of critical importance is the understanding that published guidelines, reviews, and individual study reports should not be accepted at face value, even when they are issued by professional associations or published in clinical and research journals. Reports of methodologically flawed evidence articles do get published. In addition to concerns about the trustworthiness of the research evidence, the project team or individual considering using a piece of research evidence must also determine whether the research evidence is likely to have a significant clinical **impact** and whether it is feasible for their organization to base care on them. The term **appraisal** refers to an evaluation of the value of the evidence, both its inherent value and its value to a particular user.

Appraisal is a step beyond extracting the *why, how,* and *what* of the guideline, review, or study. It involves going beyond understanding how the research evidence was produced to judge the soundness of the production methods and whether they are credible, clinically important, and applicable to a particular setting. However, it's also important to remember that appraisal as you will be doing it is not equivalent to a thesis or dissertation. Most of your time will be spent reading the evidence and marking it up for later reference. As a novice reader of research evidence, reading for true understanding and extracting essential details can be a slow go. The time required for the actual appraisal is typically much less.

Appraisal Systems

While we refer to the **Johns Hopkins model tools**, there are many other appraisal systems for evaluating the quality of guidelines, systematic reviews, and studies. Six that are widely used are listed in **Box 13-1**; their websites are listed in the *Resources* section at the end of this chapter.

These appraisal tools—and others—require considerable research knowledge to complete. The **Johns Hopkins model** appraisal guides referred to in this text are much easier for students who are encountering evidence-based practice appraisal for the first time.

Appraisal in General

The goal of critical appraisal of any type of research evidence is to systematically and thoughtfully judge whether the research evidence is:

- Credible
- Clinically significant
- Applicable

In each of the appraisal tools, there are questions specific to each area of appraisal that will help you reach a bottom-line judgment for each area and ultimately

---

Box 13-1 International Appraisal Systems

- The **AGREE II** instrument assesses the methodological rigor of how a clinical practice guideline was developed. It consists of 23 items organized within six domains, followed by two global rating items for an overall assessment.
- The **GRADE system** rates the quality of evidence in systematic reviews and guidelines about the effects of health care using four explicitly defined levels (High to Very Low), and grades the strength of recommendations in guidelines (strong and weak).
- The Institute of Medicine issued a document called Clinical Practice Guidelines We Can Trust that sets standards for developing trustworthy clinical practice guidelines (CPGs). It sets forth eight standards with several more specific standards under each main standard.
- The **PRISMA** Statement is a guide for the reporting of systematic reviews and meta-analyses but also can be used for critical appraisal of systematic reviews. It consists of a 27-item checklist and several flow diagrams.
- **CONSORT 2010** focuses on the reporting of a randomized clinical trial—how the trial was designed, analyzed, and interpreted. It consists of a 25-item checklist and a flow diagram.
- **SRQR**, Standards for reporting qualitative research is a 21-item list of standards developed by five authors.

make a decision whether the research evidence should be used as an evidence source. The following sections are a brief introduction to each appraisal domain. In Chapters 14, 15, and 16, each appraisal domain will be discussed.

Synopsis

The starting point for appraisal of all forms of research evidence is identifying why the guideline/systematic review/study was done, how it was produced, and what was found. You're on familiar ground here; this is what you learned earlier in Part 1 of this text. Actually, you could write a useful synopsis using *why, how,* and *what* as a template. In the **Johns Hopkins model appraisal tools**, you are asked more specific questions about each type of research evidence to help guide you in thinking about those three critical questions: credibility, clinical significance, and applicability.

Writing a synopsis not only ensures that you have an understanding of the evidence, but also provides a brief to refer back to later. Importantly, a synopsis contains just the facts, no judgments or interpretations. Research articles typically are very dense, meaning that every sentence contains important information; there is little fluff. Consequently, you may find that to complete the synopsis you have to refer to the article quite a few times to answer the synopsis questions.

Credibility

The central issue in appraising the **credibility** of the evidence is to make a judgment about whether the research evidence is to be trusted. If the research evidence is biased in any way, the evidence should not be trusted. **Bias** in the evidence-based practice context includes factors that influence the evidence produced in a way that is not truly objective or that distorts the truthfulness of the results. Bias can be identified in the researcher's inclinations and thinking or in the methods used. Bias is usually not intentional but rather unconscious or unrecognized by the researcher. Bias can occur during the conduct of a study while conducting a systematic review, or during the production of a clinical practice guideline.

Sometimes the bias is determined by the information reported about how the study was done, but other times it may be suspected by what was not reported or addressed. For instance, in a study comparing a post-hospital, home-based exercise program to usual care without special follow-up, the authors concluded that those who received the program had higher exercise levels at 12 weeks after discharge than those who received usual care. The report showed that the control group had almost twice the loss to follow-up of the treatment group. However, the researchers did not analyze if or how the profiles of the groups were changed by the dropouts. This lapse makes it impossible to determine if the uneven dropout rates introduced bias.

One can envision several possible ways the results might have been affected. To consider the previous example, if the dropouts in the control group were younger than the stay-ins, the average age of the control group would have been raised, which would have disrupted the original age equality of the two groups created by randomization. Thus, age could have entered as an influence on scores by making the treatment group scores look better than they would have been had all the original control group contributed outcome data. This is an example of a potential source of bias not being acknowledged by the authors and thereby bringing the credibility of the findings of this study into serious doubt. Unrecognized bias during the conduct of a study can be passed along to a systematic review, and bias at the review stage can be incorporated into the production of guidelines. Thus, it is important that appraisal be performed for each form of evidence in the credibility chain.

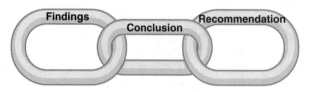

Credibility Chain

Questions to help you detect bias and to evaluate credibility chain issues are included in the **Johns Hopkins appraisal tools** suggested as a guide for you.

Clinical Significance

In general terms, clinically significant findings are those that have enough impact or importance to make a difference in patients' health outcomes or life experiences should they be used as a basis for practice. Appraising **clinical significance** would lead you to ask questions such as the following:

- Is the average increase in patients' coping abilities found in the study sizeable enough to make practical differences in patients' everyday lives?
- Are the conclusions found in a systematic review about changes in women's attitudes regarding osteoporosis prevention after education about it likely to produce a change in their dietary, exercise, or smoking behaviors?
- Are the insights reported by a systematic review with qualitative synthesis about the experience over several decades of living with a history of breast cancer after successful treatment informative enough to provide clinicians who see these women for follow-up with a fresh perspective on the care they give these women?
- Is the lower end of the 95% confidence interval around a difference in the means of an outcome variable enough of a difference that intervention A is likely to be more effective than intervention B in the population?
- Was the panel producing the evidence based clinical guideline made up of people with the necessary expertise?

In short, how robust is the evidence from a clinical perspective? Regrettably, the clinical significance of research evidence is often not explicitly discussed in research reports and guidelines. There may be a clinical implications paragraph in the discussion section, but too often this consists mainly of opinions about how the findings could be used. That is different than interpreting the results in terms of whether the difference found is clinically meaningful or, for qualitative evidence, an issue or social process uncovered is clinically informative. As a result, sometimes you will have to piece together your judgment about the clinical significance of recommendations, conclusions, and findings from what is reported in combination with your clinical knowledge. The fact that clinical significance is not always explicitly addressed is not a reason to gloss over it in appraisal; it is an important consideration.

Applicability

If the research evidence is judged credible and clinically significant, the next step is to determine whether it applies to your setting, patients, and resources. If it is not credible and clinically significant, you do not need to proceed to appraise the **applicability** because the research evidence should not be used as a basis for practice. The applicability questions that should be asked will vary depending on the form of the evidence being translated into a care protocol and the nature of the change or changes being considered. Generally, the questions fall into four categories:

1. Fit of the evidence to the setting's patients
2. Safety
3. Expected benefit
4. Feasibility of incorporating the change

Fit of the Evidence

The fit question is, "Were the persons who made up the samples of the studies similar to those in our setting?" Making a judgment regarding this fit will require taking note of the profile of persons who participated in the studies and the characteristics of the settings in which the studies were conducted. Sometimes a subgroup of patients studied will match the patients in your setting and you can pay particular attention to the evidence from that subgroup.

Safety and Expected Benefit

Safety and expected benefits are important considerations. Both safety and expected benefits must be thoughtfully considered prior to the decision to introduce a new care protocol or make a major change in practice. If a new approach to care is likely to produce meaningful benefits to patients and has few associated risks, the other hurdles can usually be overcome. The expected benefit and possible adverse events should actually be quantified. The quantification of the expected benefit is informed by what was found in the research studies. The agency can then collect data to determine if its patients achieved the expected level of benefit.

As an example, let's say a new care protocol for patient self-monitoring of blood glucose and administration of insulin is being introduced in a clinic. The goal is to have fewer patients whose blood glucose is not in the optimal range. Based on findings from the research studies and on data indicating patients' current level of control, the expected benefit might be stated as, "We expect an absolute decrease of 5% in the percentage of patients whose hemoglobin HbA1c values are above 7." Such a specific target in combination with data about the percentage of patients not meeting the target would quantify the impact of evidence based change in practice.

Feasibility

The ability of the setting to implement a clinical intervention in a way that is similar to how it was delivered in the studies or guidelines is another important consideration. If major changes must be made because of limited resources or political forces, then the question could be raised as to whether the intervention being implemented will indeed be evidence-based.

Feasibility also involves asking whether the change required could be implemented and maintained in the agency. Does it have the resources? Does it have the will? How much will it cost? The project team should consider whether their setting has the professional skills, support services, equipment, financial resources, and support of key persons to make the change and sustain it over time. A change that involves high cost or considerable effort on the part of direct care providers or support services faces an uphill road to successful implementation.

The applicability questions outlined in the guides are directed at making an organizational change in practice; that is, implementing a new approach to care. Changing individual practice would involve fewer issues; however, risk, resources needed, and people affected should still be considered.

The guides for individual studies do not include applicability questions. That is because changing clinical practice based on findings from any single study should always be undertaken with caution, particularly when the current approach to care is not causing major problems and is thought to be at least somewhat effective. The assumption is that before a change in practice is made, several studies will be considered and applicability will be appraised based on across-study conclusions, not on findings from just one original study. Analysis of findings across several studies is addressed in Chapter 16.

In summary, four domains (synopsis, credibility, clinical significance, and applicability) serve as a template for the appraisal criteria outlined in question form for the recommendations of clinical practice guidelines, for the conclusions of systematic reviews, and for the findings of original studies. The endpoint question of an appraisal is: should we use the recommendation, conclusion, or finding to develop a unit, departmental, or agency clinical change in practice?

Practical Considerations

Even though appraisal of research evidence is done using a set of objective criteria, appraisal inevitably involves a bit of judgment. Not infrequently, two appraisers using the same set of criteria will reach different judgments about the overall quality of a piece of evidence. The difference occurs for a variety of reasons, including the following:

- One appraiser may view a methodological weakness as minor, whereas the other appraiser may view it as a critical flaw that undermines the credibility of the recommendations/conclusions/findings.
- One appraiser may consider bias or failure to control confounding influences in the way a study was done to be a major detractor from its credibility, but the other appraiser may view the same circumstances as inherent in the situation.
- One appraiser may conclude that the findings of several studies are similar, while the other appraiser may see an important difference in them.

For these reasons, appraisal of a body of research evidence is most often done by two or more appraisers so that consensus can be reached or arbitrated. It's important to remember that when appraising research evidence, you have to strike a balance between identifying critical flaws and being overly critical. There is no such thing as a perfect guideline/review/study. The goal is not to identify every weakness; rather, you want to detect methods that introduce the possibility of bias to the point that they put in doubt the credibility of the end products. Ultimately, this is a judgment. When researchers design guidelines, reviews, or studies, they often have to make trade-offs between the ideal and the possible or conduct their work with limited resources. Thus, you should reject only recommendations, conclusions, or findings that were produced in a seriously flawed way. Sometimes it is a fine line between being seriously flawed and of weak-but-acceptable quality. Appraisal guides can help you make that differentiation.

Importantly, these guides require research knowledge all baccalaureate and advanced practice nurses should possess. Therefore, you should be able to answer the questions in the appraisal guides with the knowledge you acquired in reading the first part of the book and/or from your previous education and clinical experience. Importantly, using the **Johns Hopkins model** appraisal guides will help you develop basic appraisal skills to use more demanding appraisal guides in the future.

Appraisal of the three forms of research evidence are discussed in Chapters 14, 15, and 16; the guides can be accessed through the link previously shared. The same template is used for each form of research directing you to specific questions pertinent to the type of research being reviewed. The chapters are deceptively short because the real work of getting a handle on appraisal requires that you actually use the appraisal guide and that will take considerable time. Just reading the chapters will not lead to true understanding or skill in appraisal; you have to do several appraisals to begin to acquire an appreciation for what is involved.

Already Appraised Evidence

Finally, in reading articles about evidence-based practice, you may see reference to "filtered evidence." Systematic reviews and evidence-based practice guidelines are considered *filtered evidence* because, when well done, the studies and reviews incorporated in them have already been appraised for quality; the poor studies have been eliminated from the analysis. However, the systematic review or evidence-based clinical practice guideline (EbCPG) itself should also be appraised to be sure that bias did not enter during its production. An important note: if the studies in an systematic review were appraised for quality for the production of an EbCPG, they do not need to be appraised again.

Resources that summarize systematic reviews and EbCPGs along with an appraisal of their strengths and weaknesses are increasingly becoming available. One such source is the journal *Evidence-Based Nursing*; high-quality reviews and original study articles are summarized in brief commentaries that address methods, findings, and clinical application of the findings. This type of resource will be discussed at length in Chapter 19 as it is particularly useful at the point of care.

Resources

AGREE II. http://www.agreetrust.org/agree-ii/
CONSORT. http://www.consort-statement.org/
GRADE. http://www.gradeworkinggroup.org/FAQ/index.htm
Institute of Medicine. (2011). Clinical practice guidelines we can trust. http://iom.nationalacademies
    .org/Reports/2011/Clinical-Practice-Guidelines-We-Can-Trust.aspx
PRISMA. http://www.prisma-statement.org/
SRQR Standards for reporting qualitative research. (2014). http://www.mmcri.org/deptPages/core
    /downloads/QRIG/Standards_for_Reporting_Qualitative_Research___A_990451.pdf

CHAPTER 14

Appraising Recommendations of Clinical Practice Guidelines

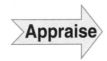

Even when a guideline carries a title indicating it is evidence-based, a measure of skepticism is needed as bias may have entered somewhere along the credibility chain and been carried forward, or it may have entered into the production of the guideline itself. Several international organizations have criteria for appraising the credibility of clinical practice guidelines: National Health and Medical Research Council, 2023; Qaseem et al., 2012; Graham et al., 2011; Registered Nurses' Association of Ontario, 2022; and Scottish Intercollegiate Guidelines Network, 2022. Generally, the appraisal standards of these organizations require a somewhat advanced level of research knowledge and are quite detailed and lengthy. The **Johns Hopkins model** appraisal tool identified as "Non-research Evidence" (located here: https://www.ijhn-education.org/node/18409#overlay-context=node/18409) includes the most important elements from these more in-depth guides and uses language appropriate to nurses with a practice-focused nursing degree. The questions in the "Non-research Evidence" appraisal guide will help you detect both transmitted and production sources of bias in guidelines. In addition, the appraisal tool will allow you to get a sense of how much clinical benefit might be expected and whether use of the guideline would be feasible in a particular setting.

Synopsis

The first step in the appraisal of a clinical practice guideline is to get a grasp of the following:

- The purpose of the guideline (health condition, intervention, population, and outcomes it addresses)
- The production process that was used
- Recommendations that were made
- System used to grade the recommendations

At this point, we suggest you look at the questions within the **Johns Hopkins model** appraisal tools. You will see that the questions in the appraisal guide ask you to extract the information just listed.

Credibility

Bias is the leading credibility issue leading to recommendations that are not truly based on sound evidence and are not likely to benefit patients. Sources of bias in the production of EbCPGs can take the following forms:

- Search for relevant evidence was not systematic and comprehensive
- Use of systematic reviews that did not eliminate studies of poor quality
- Not recognizing differences in evidence for different populations and subpopulations
- Not recognizing important differences in the interventions studied
- Downplaying or not taking into account undesirable outcomes
- Flawed judgments regarding the evidence for each recommendation

In broad terms, appraising the credibility of a guideline involves examining the following aspects of the guideline:

- Whether the organization and persons that produced the guideline had the expertise to do so
- Whether the process used to produce the guideline was systematic and free of bias
- Whether the recommendations are true to the evidence
- The confidence the developers have in the recommendations

Production Process

Ideally, the production process of the EbCPGs should be described in some detail as this allows potential adopters to determine if the guideline was produced in accord with recognized standards (Graham et al., 2011). It's important to remember that the production standards may not be in the written document. Unfortunately, some guidelines make available no or very little information about the production process. Omission of, or questionable information about, the development process makes appraising the credibility of a guideline almost impossible. Perhaps the most frequently omitted steps by developers are: (1) appraisal of the systematic reviews used to formulate the recommendations; and (2) a description or grading of the body of evidence in support of each recommendation.

Recommendations Are True to the Evidence

The supporting evidence sources should be available either in the guideline itself or in an accompanying document. Ideally, a table detailing each evidence source and a description of the body of the evidence in support of each recommendation is the best way of conveying the nature, strength, and consistency of the evidence in support of a recommendation. Often separate evidence tables are constructed for different issues; for example, evidence pertaining to one type of intervention is in one table and evidence pertaining to another intervention is in another table.

Based on the credentials of the developing organization, you can either trust the rating of the evidence or you can look into the evidence tables and description of supporting evidence to determine whether you agree with their translation and rating. We obviously favor a bit of examination of the linkage between the evidence and each recommendation. Most often we just examine the evidence tables and rarely go back to the original research reports.

Confidence in Each Recommendation

Most guidelines rate the confidence they have in their recommendations but the systems used are quite variable in terms of what is taken into account in the rating levels. Often the confidence in recommendations rating is done in addition to rating the quality and/or level of evidence. However, some recommendation rating systems combine the evidence rating into the recommendation rating system along with other considerations (as discussed in Chapter 10).

Features Indicating Soundly Developed Recommendations

- Clear guideline purposes
- Production process that included all widely recognized steps
- For each recommendation: A clear linkage between the evidence and the recommendation
- Provision of the relevant sources of evidence and a discussion of the body of evidence
- Grading of the confidence the panel has in each recommendation

Current Status

If a guideline was produced four or more years ago, it would be advisable to search for more recent research evidence that might update the recommendations of the guideline. Many guideline developers require updates every 2–3 years (Vernooij et al., 2014). Research on some clinical topics (such as management of the blood sugar levels of diabetics) is being done at a fairly fast rate; thus, a guideline or review done even two years earlier could be out of date. In contrast, other clinical topics receive much less research attention so that a guideline is stable for quite a few years.

Clinical Significance

Evaluating the clinical significance of guideline recommendations requires consideration of the following:

- Identification of essential elements of recommended action
- Magnitude of benefit associated with each recommendation
- Likelihood of benefit/outcome being realized
- Side effects and risks associated with the recommendation
- Acceptability and feasibility of the recommendation to patients
- Practicality of the recommendation in real-world practice

Consideration of these issues determines whether the recommendation would be feasible to implement and make a difference in patients' state of wellness or well-being.

To truly have clinical impact, the set of recommendations that make up the guideline should address all the issues that are important to patients as well as all the important decisions care providers make while delivering care. Some guideline developers pilot test their guidelines prior to releasing them. If this is done, it addresses the clinical significance issue by providing future users with information about how patients and providers view the value and practicality of the recommendations and whether following the guidelines is likely to result in the presumed outcome.

Applicability

Assuming that the recommendations are credible and that the producers have a reasonable level of confidence in the recommendations, the final appraisal task is to judge the fit between the recommendations and the setting in which you intend to implement them. As a student, if you are familiar with a caregiving setting, you should try to envision what would be involved in making the changes in practice that a new care protocol requires. The applicability questions will help you think through some of those requirements. At the very least, you should consider the applicability questions and appreciate what is involved in making an organizational change in care practice. The implementation of a research-based change in practice receives more attention in Chapter 17.

A guideline can be soundly produced and make credible and clinically significant recommendations. Still, it may not be feasible for the setting in which a protocol project team intends to use it. Perhaps the population of patients or providers in the setting is not similar to those for whom the guideline was intended. Perhaps the implementation of the protocol would require expenditure for training that is beyond what the setting can afford. Thus, one possible bottom-line judgment resulting from the appraisal of a guideline may be, "The guideline's recommendations are credible and clinically significant but do not apply to our setting." Alternatively, some recommendations within the clinical guideline may be applicable while others are not.

Appraisal Guide Format

The questions in the appraisal guide are stated so that a *Yes* answer indicates compliance with an appraisal criterion. Thus, a column of *Yes* answers in a domain indicates adequate quality and will undoubtedly lead you to a positive, bottom-line decision for that appraisal domain. In contrast, a mix of *Yes* and *No* answers should cause you to pause and rate the quality of the guideline appropriately. Generally, guideline recommendations are implemented as a whole, but this doesn't need to be the case. Even though the questions ask about the guideline as a whole, there may be times when you should appraise the individual recommendations separately. The most common situation in which you would do this is when the strength of evidence or confidence rating is strong for one recommendation but is weak for another.

Your Turn

Now then, it's time to reread the clinical guideline referred to in Chapter 10 about screening for Atrial Fibrillation: *Screening for Atrial Fibrillation: US Preventive Services Task Force Recommendation Statement* (Davidson et al., 2022). After re-reading, complete an appraisal of its recommendations using the questions in the Johns Hopkins model appraisal tool identified as "Non-research Evidence" (located here: https://www.ijhn-education.org/node/18409#overlay-context=node/18409). Although most questions on the appraisal guide ask for a yes/no answer, for most purposes and particularly for student learning, a one- to three-sentence rationale for the yes/no answer should be considered. For the applicability questions, assume that you work in a multi-provider primary care practice and that you do intake interviews and meet briefly with returning patients before they see their primary care provider. The practice also runs a healthy aging workshop four times a year. To get various perspectives, you might want to do the appraisal with one or several classmates.

References

Grading of Recommendations Assessment, Development and Evaluation Working Group. (n.d.). *The GRADE approach.* https://www.gradeworkinggroup.org/

Graham, R., Mancher, M., Miller Wolman, D., Greenfield, S., & Steinberg, E. (Eds.). (2011). *Clinical practice guidelines we can trust.* National Academies Press. https://doi.org/10.17226/13058

National Health and Medical Research Council. (2023). Building a healthy Australia. https://www.nhmrc.gov.au/

Qaseem, A., Forland, F., Macbeth, F., Ollenschläger, G., Phillips, S., & van der Wees, P. (2012). Guidelines International Network: Toward international standards for clinical practice guidelines. *Annals of Internal Medicine, 156*(7), 525–531. https://doi.org/10.7326/0003-4819-156-7-201204030-00009

Registered Nurses' Association of Ontario. (2022). Best practice guidelines. https://rnao.ca/bpg/guidelines

Scottish Intercollegiate Guidelines Network (SIGN). (2022). Improving patient care through evidence-based guidelines. https://www.sign.ac.uk/

Vernooij, R. W. M., Sanabria, A. J., Solà, I., Alonso-Coello, P., & García, L. M. (2014). Guidance for updating clinical practice guidelines: A systematic review of methodological handbooks. *Implementation Science, 9,* Article 3. https://doi.org/10.1186/1748-5908-9-3

CHAPTER 15

Appraising Conclusions of Systematic Reviews with Narrative Synthesis

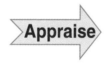

Systematic reviews are important resources when designing evidence-based care innovations. The comprehensive synthesis they provide is essential to a complete understanding of clinical topics. However, research evidence in the form of the conclusions of systematic reviews, like the recommendations of clinical practice guidelines, must be critically appraised before using them as the basis for nursing care protocols or even for the care of an individual patient. Systematic review conclusions are a bit easier to appraise than guideline recommendations because translating evidence into recommendations is not an issue. Still, there is much to consider as the move from individual to across-studies conclusions is susceptible to bias.

The appraisal framework discussed in this chapter uses the Research Appraisal tool from the Johns Hopkins model introduced in Chapter 13. The questions in the appraisal guide are specific to systematic reviews with narrative synthesis, the most common type of systematic review seen in clinical nursing journals. The systematic reviews with narrative synthesis from Chapter 9 about safety and effectiveness of parent or nurse-controlled analgesia in neonates is used to demonstrate the appraisal of an systematic reviews with narrative synthesis.

Several premier organizations have spelled out standards for conducting systematic reviews (Cochrane Training, 2017; Eden et al., 2011; Joanna Briggs Institute, 2015). The Johns Hopkins appraisal tool for systematic reviews with narrative synthesis is representative of, albeit more basic than, the criteria of the premier producers and policy setters.

Synopsis

We've already made a case for completing a synopsis of the various forms of research evidence, and we suggest completing a synopsis for systematic reviews with narrative synthesis. Recall the first step in any appraisal is to get a grasp of the following:

- The purpose of the systematic reviews with narrative synthesis.
- The production process that was used.
- Recommendations that were made.
- System used to grade the recommendations.

Credibility

Systematic reviews with narrative synthesis is prone to bias because it is all too easy for the reviewers to introduce their own predilections and beliefs into the review and synthesis process (Oxman & Guyatt, 1988). For this reason, the standards for systematic reviews with narrative synthesis include the requirements that the reviewers (1) set out the evidence from the individual studies, and (2) be explicit about how important steps in the review were done (Eden et al., 2011). This requires that systematic reviews with narrative synthesis reports include the following elements:

- A clear statement indicating the objective of the review.
- A description of how the search for relevant study reports was performed.
- A description of the criteria for including or excluding studies.
- A description of how the quality of individual studies was appraised and considered in the analysis.
- A flow diagram giving number of studies, screened, assessed for eligibility, and included in the review with reasons for exclusions (Page et al., 2021).
- Tables or narrative that describes the population, methods, and findings of the individual studies.
- For each conclusion, a clear summary of the evidence that led to it, including the quality of studies, the quantity of studies, and the consistency of findings across the supporting studies (Agency for Healthcare Research and Quality, n.d.; Eden et al., 2011).

When the research reviewers include these elements in their report, the reader is provided with information that can be used to decide if the conclusions are indeed derived from the across-studies synthesis of individual studies and are unbiased. If the reviewers do not provide this information, the reader is in the position of having to trust the reviewers' interpretation of the evidence, which is not in keeping with the explicit nature of scientific decision making.

The reviewers should be careful not to reach conclusions that are beyond what the evidence shows. This would be the case if the conclusions were applied to elders generally, but the studies had been done mainly with elders living in assisted living residences. Another example of going beyond the findings would be overstating the importance of the findings from several weak studies.

Importantly, when the evidence is inconsistent across studies or from weak studies, the reviewers should not conclude that there is no effect, no difference, or no association. Rather, the conclusion should be that definitive evidence for or against an effect or association is lacking. A conclusion of *no effect* or *no association* assumes a clear finding of no effect based on consistent evidence. In contrast, a

Recommendation	Evidence
Recommend	Sufficient, acceptable quality, and consistent
Recommend against	Sufficient, acceptable quality, and consistent
No Recommendation	Insufficient, low quality, and/or inconsistent

conclusion of *inconclusive evidence* or *insufficient evidence* recognizes that the evidence does not provide a clear and consistent answer regarding effect or association—two very different conclusions.

Clear connectivity between the findings of the individual studies and the conclusions is established when the reviewers demonstrate a deep analysis of the data. The reviewers should convince you that they looked for patterns and similarities in findings and reasons for the differences. Reasons for different findings from one study to others would include differences in the samples studied, the form of an intervention, the outcomes studied, how the variables were measured, different measurement intervals, or length of follow-up. In short, conclusions based on a deep analysis give you, the consumer of the conclusions, confidence in their credibility.

Clinical Significance

To be clinically significant, the conclusions of a review should reflect issues that are important in everyday practice and that if incorporated into practice would make a difference in patient safety, comfort, or health outcomes. For reviews of interventions, this would include a conclusion that the treatment effect is large enough to be of benefit given costs and any burden to patients or staff. This judgment is easier to make when measures of treatment effect such as absolute benefit improvement, numbers needed to treat findings, and economic analysis are provided. Clinical significance is more difficult to appraise in systematic reviews with narrative synthesis of issues other than intervention effectiveness. However, the consistency of the findings across the studies, the strength of the relationship between variables across the studies, and the informativeness of the conclusions can be considered.

Applicability

The judgment regarding whether the conclusions of a review apply to a particular setting is determined in part by the setting and patients included in the original studies reviewed. If they are similar, or the reporting is such that you can identify a subset of studies conducted in a setting similar to yours, then the results of that subset would apply to your setting. For instance, an emergency department in a rural hospital would have to consider whether the conclusions of a review about triage systems apply to its setting if all the studies included in the review were from inner-city or suburban emergency departments. The issues for the rural emergency department are very different. For instance, they are unlikely to be able to close admissions and divert ambulances elsewhere and are more likely to have fewer clinical services available 24/7. Beyond the settings and patients studied, the feasibility of implementing, the resources required, and the costs of implementing should also be taken into account.

Your Turn

We suggest that you reread the Chapter 9 exemplar study by Muirhead, Kynoch, Peacock and Lewis (2021): Safety and effectiveness of parent or nurse-controlled analgesia in neonates: A systematic review. *JBI Evidence Synthesis, 20*(1), 3–36. https://doi.org/10.11124 /JBIES-20-00385. Assume you are on a project team in a NICU examining the safety and effectiveness of parent- or nurse-controlled analgesia in neonates for the purpose of practicing your hand at appraising systematic reviews with narrative synthesis. Complete the appraisal using the *Research Evidence Appraisal Tool* (Dang et al., 2022). You could practice additional appraisals of systematic reviews with narrative synthesis by appraising one of the systematic reviews on the text's website. We suggest that readers new to appraisal not attempt an appraisal of an SR with statistical analysis.

References

Agency for Healthcare Research and Quality. (n.d.). *NGC and NQMC inclusion criteria.* https://www .ahrq.gov/gam/summaries/inclusion-criteria/index.html

Cochrane Training. (2017). For authors and MEs. Introducing Living Systematic Reviews. https://training.cochrane.org/resource/introducing-living-systematic-reviews

Dang, D., Dearholt, S., Bissett, K., Ascenzi, J., & Whalen, M. (2022). *Johns Hopkins evidence-based practice for nurses and healthcare professionals: Model and guidelines* (4th ed.). Sigma Theta Tau International.

Eden, J., Levit, L., Berg, A., & Morton, S. (Eds.). (2011). *Finding what works in health care: Standards for systematic reviews.* National Academies Press. https://doi.org/10.17226/13059

Graverholt, B., Forsetlund, L., & Jamtvedt, G. (2014). Reducing hospital admission from nursing home: A systematic review. *BMC Health Services Research, 14,* Article 36. https://doi.org /10.1186/1472-6963-14-36

Joanna Briggs Institute. (2015). *The Joanna Briggs Institute reviewers' manual 2015: Methodology for JBL scoping reviews.* http://joannabriggs.org/assets/docs /sumari/reviewersmanual-2014.pdf

Oxman, A. D., & Guyatt, G. H. (1988). Guidelines for reading literature reviews. *Canadian Medical Association Journal, 138,* 697–703.

Page, M. J., Moher, D., Bossuyt, P. M., Boutron, I., Hoffmann, T. C., Mulrow, C. D., Shamseer, L., Tetzlaff, J. M., Akl, E. A., Brennan, S. E., Chou, R., Glanville, J., Grimshaw, J. M., Hróbjartsson, A., Lalu, M. M., Li, T., Loder, E. W., Mayo-Wilson, E., McDonald, S., . . . McKenzie, J. E. (2021). PRISMA 2020 explanation and elaboration: Updated guidance and exemplars for reporting systematic reviews. *BMJ (Online), 372,* Article n160. https://doi.org/10.1136/bmj.n160

CHAPTER 16

Appraising Findings of Original Studies

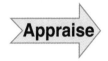

Often clinical questions or issues identified in your system have already been addressed in others. If this is the case, you may find that there are recent research-based clinical practice guidelines or systematic reviews for you to locate and appraise. In other cases, the clinical question or issue you've identified hasn't been addressed. In these situations, your team will need to appraise the findings of individual studies one at a time. A finding of a single research study is like one block or stone in a wall; it offers a contributing piece of knowledge about a topic. These individual studies often incite more questions or the need for more research, and thus, gradually more studies are done, and the knowledge about the topic becomes complete. In this chapter, we'll start with a description of how to appraise the findings of individual studies and end with a description of how to appraise findings across several studies on the same topic.

Is This a Qualitative or Quantitative Study?

The differentiation between qualitative studies and quantitative studies requires that you be able to determine which type of study you are appraising. You can identify what type of study it is by using Part 1 as a resource, using the research report to inform you, or using other resources like the list in **Box 16-1**. Knowing whether the research is qualitative or quantitative will be important to ensure you use the correct appraisal tools. For our examples, we'll use the Johns Hopkins "*Research Evidence Appraisal Tool*" available online and free for students and faculty alike (https://www.ijhn-education.org/node/18409#overlay-context=node/18409). This tool will walk you through a decision tree to identify what type of research you are appraising, and then direct you to the appropriate appraisal questions.

Box 16-1 Deciding What Type of Research Article You Are Reading

Is the study qualitative or quantitative, or was a mixed approach used?

- QuaLitative (L = language) → If the data consists of words, quotes, verbal descriptions, and/or themes, the study is a qualitative study.
- QuaNtitative (N = numbers) → If the data consists of scores, scales, numerical data, percentages, graphs, and/or statistics, the study is a quantitative study.
- Mixed Methods → If both qualitative and quantitative data are presented, the study has a mixed design.

Broad Credibility Issues

Appropriateness of Design

The credibility of findings of both qualitative and quantitative studies depends on the researcher having used study methods that were appropriate to answer the research questions. In Part 1 you read about five different research designs but were not asked to challenge whether the researcher used the right design. The study design used is determined by the question being asked. For some questions, there is not a best design, but rather several that could be good though they would provide a slightly different perspective on the question.

Let's use the example of a desire to know more about the decision-making process used by parents of a child with significant developmental delays when deciding whether to keep the child at home or place the child in residential care.

If the researcher was seeking to understand the decision-making process, a study using qualitative methods would get at the complexities of this very personal decision process and how that thinking evolves over time. The data collected would include *language* or words shared by the parents involved in the study. Alternatively, if the researcher was interested in the characteristics of families that keep a child with significant developmental delays at home, the study would use research methods that use *numbers* to quantify characteristics such as the number and ages of other children, ages of the parents, size of the extended family, social support, income, educational level, community services available, and housing situation. Such a study could produce a descriptive, quantitative profile of families who keep children with significant developmental delays at home.

If, instead of just quantifying family and community variables, the researcher wanted to explore relationships among the variables (characteristics), a correlation design could be used. For instance, if the researcher was interested in whether or not there was a relationship between the quantifiable family characteristic of community services available and the coping level of families who kept children with significant developmental delays at home, a correlational design would be appropriate. The researcher could also develop a more complex correlational design to examine multiple family and community variables to determine the best predictors of successfully keeping a child at home.

Researchers can also be interested in the differences between two groups. For instance, if the researcher wanted to know if a daycare service for children with significant developmental delays resulted in fewer children being placed in residential care than in families that were paid to take care of their child 24 hours a day, 7 days a week with only periodic paid respite, a quasi-experimental study may be best.

Peer Review

One of the most important components of credibility is whether the research report was published in a peer-reviewed journal. In general, it's assumed that research reports published in peer-reviewed journals are of higher quality than those published in journals that do not require review by peers before acceptance. This is a good assumption because peer review assures the non-researcher reader that the report has been reviewed by two or three knowledgeable persons in the field and was deemed worthy of publication. To determine if a journal is peer reviewed, you can look for a statement regarding peer review on the journal's website or in the front material of an issue of the journal. In general, the absence of a statement on the website indicating that articles are peer reviewed should raise the possibility that they are not, which should cause you to be particularly careful in your appraisal of the study's credibility.

Appraisal of the Findings of a Qualitative Study

Credibility

When considering the credibility of the findings of a qualitative study, the main consideration is the **rigor** of the study's methods. Criteria for rigor of qualitative studies come in the form of checklists, guidance from individual journals, and guidance from experienced authors and researchers in the field. Unlike quantitative research, researchers who use qualitative methodology for their studies argue that the rigor of qualitative research must remain flexible to some degree to align with the understanding that there is diversity within perspectives inherent to qualitative research (Johnson et al., 2020). Nonetheless, as a student or working nurse, you can assume that in general, the findings and interpretations of qualitative studies can be considered credible by using Glassick's criteria as a guide (Johnson et al., 2020):

- Purpose: The research has a clear purpose.
- Preparation: The research had adequate preparation including a thorough literature review and review of previous work.
- Methods: The research methodology aligns with the research question.
- Results: The results advance the knowledge and/or understanding of a targeted field of practice.
- Translation: The results are presented in a way that can be replicated and/or built on by other researchers.
- Reflective critique: There is adequate interaction between the data collection and data analysis.

Clinical Significance

The purpose of qualitative research is to expand the understanding of an individual or group's lived experience through their own perspectives, observations, experiences, or events. These perspectives, observations, experiences, and events then inform conceptual frameworks or contribute to developing new theories or models. A vivid portrayal of the experience or situation and a description of how context or events produce variations to the experience adds to the usefulness of the findings. As you read more qualitative studies, you will see that some studies capture the experience or situation and produce new insights. In contrast, others fail to get much beyond what most healthcare professionals in the field of practice already know. In brief, the clinical significance of qualitative findings pertains to their usefulness for healthcare professionals.

Applicability

As explained earlier, appraisal questions are not offered for applicability because generally an organization should not base care on the results of one study. However, the results of a single qualitative study may make a nurse more sensitive to patient experiences and preferences and may be used to fine tune their interpersonal approaches to assessment, patient teaching, and anticipatory guidance (Coleman, 2022). The usefulness of the findings from single qualitative studies is derived from the fact that most qualitative researchers provide considerable detail about the study participants' thoughts and feelings, their experiences, and the contexts of their lives. Thus, it is often quite clear with whom or in what kind of situation the findings might add insight to care.

Appraisal of the Findings of a Quantitative Study

Credibility

In quantitative studies the end products of the study are typically several related findings, which are the researchers' data-based conclusions. Like all human conclusions, they can be right, wrong, and everything in between. In correlational and experimental studies, there are two possible correct conclusions and two possible conclusion errors.

The correct conclusions include:

1. Concluding that a relationship or difference exists in the population when in reality it actually does exist.
2. Concluding that no relationship or difference exists in the population when in reality it does not exist.

The two types of **conclusion errors** include:

1. Concluding that a relationship or difference exists in the population when in reality it does not exist (**type 1 conclusion error**).
2. Concluding that no relationship or difference exists in the population when in reality it does exist (**type 2 conclusion error**).

For a graphic of these possibilities, see **Table 16-1**.

Table 16-1 Reaching Correct Conclusion

		Does a real difference exist?	
		Yes	**No**
Researcher's conclusion	Real difference	Correct	Type 1 error
	No difference	Type 2 error	Correct

Avoiding Conclusion Error

The researcher aims for correct conclusions and tries to avoid making conclusion **errors** by:

- Eliminating chance variation as an explanation.
- Avoiding low statistical power.
- Controlling for extraneous variables.
- Controlling for bias.

Chance variation, which is always present to some degree when data is collected, can affect the statistical results of a study and lead to conclusion errors. The researcher controls the role of chance variation by defining its limits. This is what is done when the researcher sets the maximal acceptable decision point *p*-level for significance at 0.05 or 0.01. In so doing, they in essence are saying, "I will accept only a low probability that my conclusion of a significant difference is due to chance variation." This in effect reduces the likelihood of a type 1 conclusion error.

Studies with small sample sizes can have statistical results indicating no relationship or effect when in fact the problem is that the sample size was not large enough (type 2 conclusion error). A too-small sample size results in insufficient statistical power to detect a significant difference. In other words, when there is insufficient data or data points, the statistical analysis is not able to detect a relationship or a difference amid the chance variation that is inevitably present. Using power analysis to determine sample size protects against type 2 conclusion errors. If you need a refresher on power analysis, head to Chapter 7 for assistance!

Other aspects of the study also determine whether a conclusion is right or wrong. As you learned earlier, researchers use inclusion/exclusion criteria, random assignment, adherence to study protocols, and awareness of what is going on in the research setting to eliminate or isolate the influence of the extraneous variables. However, it may not be possible to control all extraneous variables, or the researcher may not have thought to control a particular influence. Some extraneous variables enter a study without the researcher's awareness in the form of an event or change in the research setting, whereas still others are introduced by the research activities themselves.

Uncontrolled extraneous variables distort study results by mixing with the study variables and producing a statistical result that is an illusion. For example, a statistical result of a study may indicate that there is a significant difference in the outcomes of two treatment groups. Thus, the researcher would conclude that the experimental treatment was more (or less) effective than the control treatment. However, if the control group had considerably more people with multiple comorbidities that may alter the effect of the intervention, that might be what caused the difference in outcomes, not the difference in treatments they received. In this example, the higher number of comorbidities in the one group is an extraneous variable that could cause a difference in outcomes and lead the researcher to make a type 1 conclusion error. Statistical analysis works the numbers and does not shed any light on what caused the difference. The study design is what controls, eliminates, or identifies possible extraneous variables.

Extraneous variables can produce an illusion of a difference in effectiveness as in the example just given or an illusion of no difference in effectiveness when indeed there would have been one had the extraneous variable not been at work (i.e., type 2 conclusion error). In short, when evaluating the credibility of findings, you want to ask, "Was there anything else that could have produced the results obtained other than what the researcher concluded?" Said differently: "Is there any alternative explanation for the difference found or not found?"

Bias can enter a study at various points in the form of preconceived ideas about what the results will be or unconscious preference for one treatment over another. Bias is also a potential source of erroneous conclusions. In quantitative studies, bias is controlled by research methods such as random sampling, random assignment, checks on adherence to research protocols, blinding of study observers and/or staff, and use of placebo treatments. Generally, researchers will not speak to bias in their reports; rather, you as the reader have to be alert to the possibility of it and decide whether adequate means were taken to prevent bias from affecting study results, findings, and conclusions.

Credible Versus Valid

The appraisal questions in the Johns Hopkins *"Research Evidence Appraisal Tool"* should assist you in identifying possible sources of wrong conclusions. When the researcher's conclusions are trusted as the best explanation for the results, not chance, extraneous variables, low statistical power, or bias, the findings are deemed credible (Dang et al., 2022).

Although throughout this book the term *credible* has been used to convey that the researcher's conclusions are likely to be trustworthy, other appraisal guides ask, "Are the findings valid?" When used to characterize findings from a study, *valid* means that the findings are judged to be trustworthy reflections of reality and not the result of how the study was conducted or the result of an extraneous variable at work. Note that this usage of the word *valid* is a bit different from how it was used to characterize measurement instruments. The term *valid* is more technical and more complex than the word *credible*. However, the word *credible* has a more common-sense resonance and is an adequate substitute.

Clinical Significance

The clinical significance of the findings of a quantitative study is determined by the strength of the relationship between variables in correlational studies or the size of the difference in the outcomes of the two treatment groups in experimental or quasi-experimental studies. In a correlational study, one would consider the size of the r^2s, whereas in a study comparing interventions, one would consider

(1) the difference in the means of the two groups; (2) the absolute benefit increase; (3) the numbers needed to treat; or (4) the relative risk. Therefore, in intervention studies, the clinical significance question is: "Is the treatment effect found in the study large enough to make a clinical difference in patient outcomes or well-being?"

Applicability

Having stated the general principle that findings from a single study should not be used as the basis for a change in practice, an exception would be when a diligent search did not come up with another study and the basis for current practice is clearly not effective. Of course, the study should have been soundly conducted and the setting and sample should be similar to the patient group with whom the findings will be used. In the rare case when the findings of a single study will be used as the basis for practice, the applicability questions from the systematic review appraisal guide can be used.

Your Turn

At this point, we suggest you appraise the Chapter 7 exemplar study by Erdogan and Aytekin Ozdemir (2021). The effect of three different methods on venipuncture pain and anxiety in children: Distraction cards, virtual reality, and Buzzy® (randomized controlled trial). *Journal of Pediatric Nursing, 58*, e54–e62. https://doi.org/10.1016/j.pedn.2021.01.001 using the Johns Hopkins *"Research Evidence Appraisal Tool."*

You should also consider completing an appraisal of the Semple, McCaughan, Beck, and Hanna (2021) qualitative study in Chapter 4 or one of the qualitative studies listed on the text's website to get some practice appraising qualitative studies. The more appraisals you do, the better you will get at using the questions to make a judgment regarding the credibility and clinical significance of study findings.

Systematic Review

Now that you have some skill in appraising individual studies, you need to at least be aware of what is involved in appraising several studies regarding a question or issue. This would have to be done when an agency team could not locate an evidence-based clinical practice guideline or systematic review, but did find several relevant studies. In addition to appraising each study separately, the several studies should be appraised as a body of studies; doing so is called **systematic review** (Sutton, 2019). This will require identifying, retrieving, and appraising studies, then bringing together the findings from all relevant and sound studies.

Doing an across-studies review and summary is not something an individual should do. It is an advanced skill and is best done by a group in which the individual members' interpretations and thinking regarding the findings of the various studies can complement and correct one another. Generally, project teams who do across-studies analysis have a few members with master's or doctoral education. You may, however, be asked to be a member of an evidence-based practice (EBP) project team, in which case you will learn by direct observation how across-studies analysis is done. To prepare you for that, we offer a brief description of what across-studies analysis involves.

The goal in looking at a body of evidence is to answer the question, "What findings earn our confidence because they are well supported by one or more sound studies?" To answer this question, the protocol development team must determine the following:

- How many studies addressed the issue?
- Were the studies of good quality?
- Was the finding consistently produced by several well-conducted studies?
- If an intervention was studied, was the size of the treatment effect or the relationship of similar magnitude across the studies?
- Can inconsistencies regarding a finding be explained by study differences in patient populations or research methods?

Thus, the essential across-studies issues are the quality, quantity, and consistency of evidence across studies. If the project team is appraising two or more studies, they should work with a findings table (see **Table 16-2**). If the clinical issue has several sub-issues, such as prevention and management, the team might use separate findings tables for each sub-issue. The team may also decide to weight studies with strong methodology or samples similar to their own population of patients more heavily than studies with weak methodology or samples that are very different.

Unlike the findings of single studies, for which the general recommendation was made that they not be used as the basis for clinical protocols, whenever clear conclusions are produced by a systematic review, the conclusions can be used as the basis for practice. Appraisal of findings from several or many studies involves decisions about the credibility, clinical significance, and applicability of the body of evidence. Ideally, these decisions should be reached in a deliberative way by the consensus of the EBP project team (Dang et al., 2022). A deliberative process requires the following:

- Clear objectives.
- Careful extraction of information from reports by at least two persons.
- Clear criteria for appraising the evidence.
- Clear rules regarding how to handle studies of poor quality.
- Good analytical thinking.
- Broad participatory dialogue.
- Formal polling to resolve differences of opinion.
- Skillful chairing.

The Three-Legged Stool

Strong research evidence that has a good fit in the implementation setting is more persuasive than weaker evidence, but even strong research evidence by itself is not sufficient. While research evidence should weigh heavily in considering how to implement a change in practice, clinical experience, internal system and outcomes data, and the patient experience are also relevant forms of evidence which should also be considered.

Table 16-2 Findings Table

Author(s) and date	Questions, variables, objectives, hypotheses	Design, sample, setting	Findings	Notes
Topic			Date	

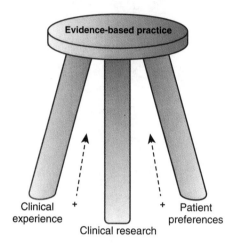

Three-legged evidence-based practice stool

Reproduced from American Career College. (n.d.). *What is evidence-based practice?* https://guides.americancareercollege.edu/c.php?g=393192&p=2673709

Wrap-Up

Evaluating a body of findings from individual studies is definitely the long and labor-intensive way of establishing the state of the science regarding an issue. However, sometimes a project group will have to do it. If necessary, it is important that the group include a person with knowledge of research methodology as a part of the EBP project team.

References

Coleman, P. (2022). Validity and reliability within qualitative research for the caring sciences. *International Journal of Caring Sciences, 14*(3), 2041–2045.

Dang, D., Dearholt, S., Bissett, K., Ascenzi, J., & Whalen, M. (2022). *Johns Hopkins evidence-based practice for nurses and healthcare professionals: Model and guidelines* (4th ed.). Sigma Theta Tau International.

Erdogan, B., & Aytekin Ozdemir, A. (2021). The effect of three different methods on venipuncture pain and anxiety in children: Distraction cards, virtual reality, and Buzzy® (randomized controlled trial). *Journal of Pediatric Nursing, 58*, e54–e62. https://doi.org/10.1016/j.pedn.2021.01.001

Johnson, J., Adkins, D., & Chauvin, S. (2020). A review of the quality indicators of rigor in qualitative research. *American Journal of Pharmaceutical Education, 84*(1), 138–146.

Semple, C. J., McCaughan, E., Beck, E. R., & Hanna, J. R. (2021). "Living in parallel worlds"— bereaved parents' experience of family life when a parent with dependent children is at end of life from cancer: A qualitative study. *Palliative Medicine, 35*(5), 933–942. https://doi.org/10.1177/02692163211001719

Sutton, A., Clowes, M., Preston, L., & Booth, A. (2019). Meeting the review family: exploring review types and associated information retrieval requirements. *Health Information and Libraries Journal, 36*, 202–222.

CHAPTER 17

Evidence-Based Practice Strategies

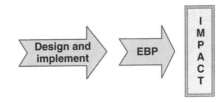

In Part 1 we introduced you to different types of research evidence; in Part 2 we've presented how to appraise the quality of the evidence, and in this chapter, we begin the next phase of evidence-based practice—translation into practice.

Strategies for Translation

The road from the conduct of research to healthcare providers using evidence to inform their care practice is lengthy. While there are multiple reasons for this "gap" between research and implementation into practice, using evidence-based practice models to guide implementation within systems can help to reduce both the time to translation and the potential for healthcare waste for unnecessary practice(s). There is an entire field of research called translational science that explores implementation interventions, factors, and other contextual variables that affect knowledge uptake and use in practices and communities (Titler, 2018). This research has led to multiple evidence-based practice implementation models and theories that can be used in translating evidence to practice such as the Promoting Action on Research Implementation in Health Services (PARIHS)/i-PARIHS model (Harvey & Kitson, 2016), the Diffusion of Innovation Theory (Dearing, 2009), the Iowa Model of EBP to Improve the Quality of Care (Iowa Model Collaborative, 2017), and the Johns Hopkins Nursing Evidence-Based Practice Model (Johns Hopkins model).

The Johns Hopkins Nursing Evidence-Based Practice Model

We've chosen the Johns Hopkins model for its ease of use, its foundational understanding that evidence-based practice is a cyclical process that doesn't have any "final steps," and its acknowledgment that while EBP always happens within the confines of a team, nurses can and should be leaders in this process (Dang et al., 2022). This model is based on three key factors: Inquiry, Practice, and Learning. In a fast-paced healthcare environment, it is all too common for nurses and other healthcare professionals to check off the tasks on their to-do lists without stepping back to ask whether or not there is a better or different way of approaching the task. For instance, when teaching clinical to pre-licensure students, nursing faculty often say, "You are correct; those are the steps to the task that is required for this patient, but **why** are you needing to perform the task?" Having the student step back and contemplate the approach to care with **why** instead of **how** reframes the work with what the National League for Nursing (NLN) dubs "a spirit of inquiry." As faculty, we also call this a desire or passion for lifelong learning, one of the key factors in the Hopkins model (**Figure 17-1**).

The Johns Hopkins model has 20 steps. This may seem like a lot, but you've already learned how to do the bulk of these steps in the previous chapters. Pulling that work together into an intentional project is the exciting part of EBP.

1. Recruit an EBP team.
2. Determine responsibility for project leadership.
3. Schedule team meetings.
4. Clarify and describe the problem (Chapter 11).
5. Develop and refine the EBP question (Chapter 11).
6. Determine the need for an EBP project (Chapter 11).
7. Identify stakeholders.
8. Conduct external and internal search for evidence (Chapter 12).
9. Appraise the level and quality of each piece of evidence (Chapters 13–16).

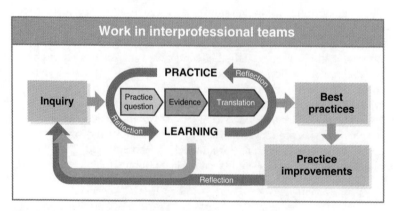

Figure 17-1 Johns Hopkins Model

Reproduced from Dang, D., Dearholt, S., Bissett, K., Ascenzi, J., & Whalen, M. (2022). *Johns Hopkins evidence-based practice for nurses and healthcare professionals: Model and guidelines* (4th ed.). Sigma Theta Tau International.

10. Summarize the individual evidence (Chapters 13–16).
11. Synthesize the findings.
12. Develop best evidence recommendations.
13. Identify practice setting–specific recommendations
14. Create an action plan.
15. Secure resources and support to implement the plan.
16. Implement the action plan.
17. Evaluate outcomes to determine whether improvements were made.
18. Report results to stakeholders.
19. Identify next steps.
20. Disseminate findings.

In the Johns Hopkins model, translating evidence into practice is the last piece of the PET process (Practice-Evidence-Translation) (Dang et al., 2022). Translation of evidence to practice is specifically associated with steps 13 through 20, which we'll walk you through over the next several pages. Before we do that, let's do a quick walkthrough of steps 1–12.

Recruiting an EBP Team

There isn't one perfect approach to recruiting an EBP team (step 1); however, the most critical component of recruitment is making sure that the team is representative of all professionals who may be influenced or have an influence on the evidence-based practice project. Keeping the group small but representative will allow for easier scheduling of meetings.

Leadership

Identifying a leader within the team to facilitate the EBP change is critical to the team's success (step 2). The adoption of a change is correlated to a leader's involvement, attitude, and commitment toward that change, as well as the leader's ability to engender the establishment of a team mission, vision, and collective accountability to the change process. Importantly the team should represent all stakeholders in the proposed change and have a broad skill set including operational knowledge of how the clinical processes and support systems of the setting work; sensitivity to the characteristics of the recipients and their current way of doing things; knowledge about how to appraise and translate research evidence into setting-specific protocols; and skill in working collaboratively with management and opinion leaders in the system into which the evidence-based practice change will be introduced.

Scheduling Meetings

These days, finding time and space for meeting (step 3) may be a bit easier due to the expansion of virtual meeting space. During your first meeting, you'll want to create team norms and rules. This is a critical first step to working in any team to assure accountability from all members, to clarify expectations and, perhaps most importantly, to eliminate the challenges of miscommunication halfway through a project when teamwork is critical.

Clarifying, Developing, and Determining Need

Lucky for you, all you need to do is head back to Chapter 11 for steps 4–6 and you'll be set!

Identifying Stakeholders

To facilitate the implementation of evidence-based practice, the project team facilitating the implementation must identify the persons who will be affected (step 7). The stakeholders must truly understand how they will be affected by the proposed change and be involved in each step. Stakeholders should be viewed as individuals and a community of practice, that is, all nurses working on the unit or in a department such as respiratory therapy. Active involvement of the end users of the change has been shown to lead to greater acceptance and adoption of the required actions (Harrison et al., 2013). If you aren't sure who your stakeholders are, the following questions can assist you:

1. Who asked for the project?
2. Who will use the product/service/change that is being created or enhanced?
3. Who will have to change the way they do their jobs because of the project?
4. Who has the authority to make decisions about the project?
5. Who can give or take away resources from the project?
6. Who has an influence on or over those who will make decisions about the project?

After you've identified your initial list of stakeholders, the next part is getting a sense of what their interests and needs are. This should generally be done early on in the project development. Once you've gathered all this information, the next step is the analysis. Analyzing your stakeholders will help you to determine where to focus your time and energy since it's feasible that you may have more stakeholders than you can possibly attend to. One way to do this is through the use of a power and interest grid (image).

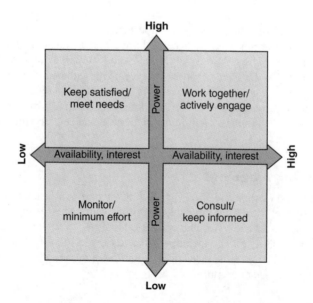

Using a power and interest grid helps you to identify which stakeholders have an interest in your project and which ones have the most potential to drive your project to success. These are the stakeholders that you want to focus your attention on! For instance, if someone has low interest and high power, you want to keep them satisfied with the project. If someone has low interest and low power, you want to keep in touch with them and monitor their involvement to ensure that they do not begin to take a negative view of the project. If someone has high interest and low power, you want to make sure that you keep them informed of the project status. The stakeholders you want to focus the majority of your time and attention on are those with high interest and high power.

Another way to think of the types of stakeholders via your power and interest grid is through the terms promoters, defenders, latents, and apathetics. *Promoters* have both great interest in the effort and the power to help make it successful (or to derail it). *Defenders* have a vested interest and can voice their support in the community, but have little actual power to influence the effort in any way. *Latents* have no particular interest or involvement in the effort but have the power to influence it greatly if they become interested, and *Apathetics* have little interest and little power, and may not even know the effort exists.

Now that you've done your analysis and know where you're going to focus your time and energy, the next step is figuring out a means of "managing" your stakeholders. A critical part of managing your stakeholders involves understanding what information they need, and when they need it. You also want to consider how they need it. Not everyone wants an email or a text; some people prefer a phone call while others would like face-to-face discussions. When possible, you want to try to work with those preferences. As your project continues to unfold, you will continue to learn more and your relationships with your stakeholders will continue to evolve. This all brings about new information that may necessitate altering your approach.

Conducting, Collecting, and Appraising

These are, by far, some of the most time-consuming steps of the model. Regardless of which model or process you end up using in your own practice, the efforts you put into these steps impact the quality of your evidence, which subsequently impacts the impacts, outcomes, and overall buy-in that your project will have. Head back to Chapters 12–16 to refresh your memory for steps 8–10.

Synthesizing and Recommending

The process of synthesizing (step 11) all the work you've done in your team to appraise the evidence you've gathered is a skill that you will continue to grow into. One of the most important aspects to remember is that synthesizing is not the same as summarizing. A summary of the literature is a shortened version of an article that highlights key points author by author. Conversely, a synthesis is taking those key points of each article and arranging them into related themes. In other words, a synthesis is a narrative of different subtopics woven together to provide a better understanding of the state of the knowledge on the larger issue or topic. For your evidence-based practice project, you may find it helpful to use a matrix to organize all the evidence you've collected and then look for themes from there— doing this through a platform like Google Docs or other shared media will allow team members to actively contribute throughout. Look for recurrent themes across your research evidence and non-research evidence such as clinical guidelines, expert opinion, or patient perspective. Identifying the level of evidence can also be helpful when it comes to getting buy in. Translation science experts suggest that for organizational level change, the use of systematic reviews and evidence-based clinical practice guidelines to effect change are more likely to be supported due to the dependable body of findings and the advantages of a credible association having summarized and translated the evidence (Titler, 2018).

Once you've synthesized your evidence, the next step (12) is forming a recommendation. This recommendation must be aligned with the system in which the change is planned (step 13). Doing so will increase the odds of success. After the clinical question has been posed, the literature reviewed, and the evidence synthesized, healthcare teams must be able to translate these findings into recommendations for practice. The following factors, in addition to the cumulative evidence reviewed, must be considered when making recommendations:

1. The risk or potential risk to the patient or patient groups the change impacts,
2. The feasibility of making the change within the practice setting (i.e., factors such as budget and space), and
3. The need for education/protocols to assure uniform adoption of the recommendation.

As an example, if you asked the clinical question "Is the Finnegan Neonatal Abstinence Scoring Tool or the Neonatal Narcotic Withdrawal Index a better evaluation for infants experiencing neonatal withdrawal following delivery?" your recommendation would need to include current practice, implications for neonatal outcomes, implications for the neonate, family, and nursing staff if a change was made, be relevant to the acute care setting immediately post birth, and consider questions like leadership support, the professional culture in the care system, resources available, financial constraints, and needed time, efforts, and other resources for a practice change.

Creating a Plan and Securing Resources

You've likely heard the old adage from Einstein "Insanity is doing the same thing over and over again and expecting different results." Creating an action plan and ensuring that you have the resources to implement your plan will improve the potential success of your project. To create an action plan, Dang et al. (2022) outline four critical components:

1. Development of any policies, procedures, pathways or processes to facilitate implementation of the change you've identified;
2. Identifying a timeline for implementation;
3. Identifying team members responsible for each implementation task/process/ phase; and
4. Checking back with those stakeholders you identified in step 7 to make sure you've got a plan that is going to work.

Protocol Formats. EBP changes often take the form of care protocols, which are developed in diverse formats: standardized plans of care, standardized order sets, **care bundles**, decision algorithms, care maps, clinical pathways, policies, and procedures. References for each of these are listed on the text's website. By way of definition, a care bundle is a group of evidence-based interventions related to a condition or treatment—generally three to five—that, when consistently performed together, result in improved patient outcomes (Institute for Healthcare Improvement, 2015). There are bundles for central line care, urinary catheter insertion and maintenance, reducing admissions for chronic obstructive pulmonary disease, and preventing sepsis, pressure ulcers, and falls, to name just a few. In ICUs, the ABCDE bundle is being used to prevent and manage ICU-acquired delirium and weakness that result from prolonged mechanical ventilation and oversedation (Marra, Ely, Pandharipande, & Patel, 2017). Based on the best available evidence, it involves coordinated awakening and breathing trials and early mobility. It is a complex clinical protocol to implement but one that produces a considerable benefit to patients.

Decision algorithms are step-by-step instructions for reaching a decision or solving a problem; they are often formatted as a flow chart consisting of a series of yes/no questions leading to one of several possible decisions or actions. An great example of the use of an algorithm can be found in a readable and practical article about the assessment and management of persistent pain in older adults (Jablonski, DuPen & Ersek, 2011).

A clinical pathway, also called a care map, is a multidisciplinary specification of the actions to be implemented during the process of care for a well-defined group of patients over a specified period of time (Lawal et al., 2016). A pathway explicitly sets forth key elements and sequences of care, time-specific goals, and specification of performance and coordinating roles.

Although some decisions and actions in decision algorithms and clinical pathways will be based on high-quality, strong research evidence, others may be based on weaker evidence such as expert opinion. The ideal is that a companion document summarizing or grading the research evidence about the decision points and recommended actions is available to clinicians.

Action!

Now it's that time to do something (step 16)! We've finally gotten back to that translation piece. One of the questions a team must ask themselves is whether the change is one that can be done within an independent evidence-based practice project in, say, one singular unit or whether the scale is larger and system wide. In either approach, the use of something called the Plan-Do-Study-Act (PDSA) cycle can help you do a "trial run" to identify any quirks or gaps in your action plan. The PDSA cycle is one model used widely within quality improvement (QI).

What Is Quality Improvement?

Let's talk first about the history of quality improvement (QI) and then how QI and EBP work together. The Centers for Medicare and Medicaid Services (CMS, 2021) define QI as:

> the framework used to systematically improve care. Quality improvement seeks to standardize processes and structure to reduce variation, achieve predictable results, and improve outcomes for patients, healthcare

systems, and organizations. Structure includes things like technology, culture, leadership, and physical capital; process includes knowledge capital (e.g., standard operating procedures) or human capital (e.g., education and training). (para. 2)

And where quality is defined as:

the degree to which health services for individuals and populations increase the likelihood of desired health outcomes and are consistent with current professional knowledge. (para. 1)

All health systems are mandated by third-party payers, such as the CMS, and by accreditors such as The Joint Commission, to provide documentation showing that the health services they provide are safe, effective, and cost-efficient. To achieve these goals, organizations collect data about their:

- Activities of care (what is being done);
- Processes of care (how it is done: when, where, by whom);
- Patient outcomes achieved
- Patient safety (low levels of adverse events in care environments);
- Patient satisfaction; and
- Cost.

History of Quality Improvement in the United States

In 1998 under a presidential directive, the quality interagency coordination task force was established requiring that all federal agencies that were involved in purchasing, providing, studying or regulating healthcare services were working together in a coordinated manner toward the common goal of improving quality care (Eisenberg et al., 2001). As this task force began to meet, the Institute of Medicine (IOM) was well underway in publishing a report highlighting the number of medical errors in U.S. hospital systems leading to mortality each year. This report, published in 1999 contributed significantly to the development of public-private partnership by the agency for healthcare research and quality and the national quality forum. This partnership had a very specific agenda: to protect patients from experiencing adverse events from exposure to the healthcare system across a variety of diseases and procedures.

In 2001, the IOM published *Crossing the Quality Chasm* emphasizing that marginal reforms similar to those that had already been initiated would be inadequate to address the systematic flaws that were prominent throughout health care. National efforts to address the glaringly ineffective, inefficient, and unsafe practices were initiated. The Joint Commission (JCAHO) led one of these efforts to address the quality gap by establishing specific standards for patient safety required of all accredited hospitals. These standards are updated each year to reflect ongoing challenges. Additional measures to address patient safety by creating hospital-wide patient safety programs are now a requirement of systems as a part of their accreditation process and approval. Despite these initiatives, there is still much work to be done.

Three specific categories of problems have received the most attention when it comes to challenges within health systems; one, underuse of beneficial services; two, overuse of procedures that are not medically necessary or warranted; and three, mistakes leading to patient injury or death (Kohn et al., 2000). To provide a framework for tackling this important work, the Institute for Healthcare Improvement (IHI) launched the Triple Aim initiative in 2007 (Berwick et al., 2008).

The first aim is one that initially might not appear to directly relate to reducing the number of adverse events; however, **improving the patient experience of care** is much larger than simply getting better patient satisfaction scores. Within this aim, there is a focus on patient safety, greater adherence to evidence-based practice, and last but not of least importance, higher patient satisfaction with the care they receive. The second aim, **improving the health of populations,** recognizes that simply improving a *sub-population* within the larger population is not adequate. All individuals deserve the highest quality of care that is safe, trustworthy, and based on evidence. The third aim calls us to **reduce the per capita cost of health care.** We doubt anyone is immune to experiencing the incredible costs associated with receiving care today and that these costs aren't always reflective of care that you would deem as excellent. Our newsfeeds are rife with stories of individuals who, without certain government-sponsored healthcare plans, would not be able to afford care and/or would not be alive because the care they needed would have been denied otherwise.

Analysis of this data and the performance improvement actions that accompany it most often go under the rubric QI. Data collection is key to QI at several points to identify problems, establish baseline performance, determine whether change made has led to improvements, and compare a health service system's outcome to other organizations providing the same service. To evaluate systems of care, QI teams examine in detail processes such as patients' timely access to services, patient movement through a health service system, the patient experience of care, staff performance of key clinical actions, coordination of care, sequence of work, availability and functionality of equipment, and who does what when.

QI Models

There are several QI models in use in health care that go by various names, including total quality management and the continuous quality improvement model (Health Resources and Services Administration [HRSA], 2022). The Plan-Do-Study-Act (PDSA) cycle we mentioned previously is one that is widely used. The PDSA cycle has four stages:

- **Plan:** Determine goals for a process and needed changes to achieve them.
- **Do:** Implement the changes.
- **Study:** Evaluate the results in terms of performance.
- **Act:** Standardize and stabilize the change or begin the cycle again, depending on the results.

Source: https://www.ahrq.gov/health-literacy/improve/precautions/tool2b.html

Other widely used quality improvement models in health care are *Six Sigma*, *Lean*, and *Root Cause Analysis*.

Evidence-Based Practice and Quality Improvement

Sometimes QI and EBP are viewed separately, but EBP is often used in QI. Research provides the evidence to inform practice where evidence-based practice is often used in QI to improve the processes and outcomes of care. This process is oversimplifying the often complex work of changing practice. Evidence-based protocols lose effectiveness if the **delivery systems** in which they are embedded are not safe, efficient, and patient-centered. While there are distinct differences between research, EBP, and QI, they are intended to work synergistically together.

Research is the intentional, systematic investigation to validate and refine existing knowledge and generate new knowledge (Gray et al., 2017).

Quality improvement is the systematic and continuous actions leading to measurable improvement in health care and the health status of populations (HRSA, 2022).

Evidence-based practice is a problem-solving approach to decision-making that searches for the best and latest evidence, clinical expertise, and patient preferences/values within the context of caring (Melynk & Fineout-Overholt, 2019).

Evaluate

Even when an evidence-based project was carefully developed and introduced, checks on its uptake and ultimate impact are necessary (step 17). If the introduction was part of a larger QI project, evaluation will naturally be undertaken. The measurements used to analyze the care system at baseline often can be repeated to determine if the change has been adopted and is having the desired impact.

Typically, measurement of performance and outcomes before, during, and after implementing a change in practice is needed to be sure that the new protocol has resulted in the desired patient outcomes and that the change is being maintained over time. After all, change is only change if it's sustained! Once you've gathered your data, share it with your stakeholders (step 18). Refer back to your stakeholder analysis to determine what your stakeholder preferences are for communication. Keeping your stakeholders in the loop is part of the evidence-based practice process.

Next Steps

If the anticipated results aren't realized, the project team may need to reexamine the context in which it was embedded, evaluate why the change wasn't effective, and determine next steps (step 19). Questions the team can ask include:

- Was the evidence not interpreted correctly?
- Was the translation of the evidence into the agency protocol faulty?
- Was the implementation lacking in some way?
- Is the protocol unrealistic or in conflict with other job expectations?

The pursuit of quality care is indeed demanding and ongoing.

Dissemination

The last step in the Johns Hopkin's model is dissemination. So often this step is overlooked, contributing to the research to practice gap. Spreading change can be a simple process, or in some cases a more complex process. Whether the process is simple or complex, a short time frame or long, largely depends on what the change is that is being adopted and always requires steadfast leadership. Whether you're a practicing nurse or are just beginning your professional career as a nurse it's important to understand the implications that exist if we don't share our knowledge. If we don't step up to the plate and take the lead questioning how, why, when, and for whom we do what we do, then our practices will remain static and our patient care will suffer.

Spreading change means using your voice, or the collective voice of a team to share what you know with others. When it comes to evidence-based practice it may feel that a change that your team initiated within your unit or organization isn't relevant to external populations—but they could be—and what a gift to give others to not have to "figure it out for themselves" but rather, to have a blueprint of sorts from which to launch and navigate the particular nuances of their own system from a great starting point! Sharing what we know, what we do, and how we do it is essential to keeping quality at the forefront of the work we do—this is true for everything from orientation best practices to best practices for the most complicated of procedures. We have nothing to gain in keeping this evidence to ourselves! Dang et al. (2022) offer an excellent template for publishing an evidence-based practice project, and we encourage you to consider doing so.

A Note on Innovation, Change, and Evidence-Based Practice

Innovation is a buzzword that you'll likely have heard at some point in time whether in your day-to-day life or within the context of the systems in which you work. Peter Drucker, an expert in innovation management, is quick to point out that novelty does not equate to innovation nor is innovation just doing something differently. Innovation is "the effort to create purposeful, focused change in an enterprise's economic or social potential" (Drucker, 2002). In short, innovation is what differentiates you from your competition; innovation is what gives you a competitive advantage that can't be easily copied by your competitors, and innovation is what ultimately has the opportunity to affect bottom-line results. EBP has a place *with* innovation but should not be confused with or equated to innovation (Weberg & Davidson, 2019).

Information Technology[1]

Implementing the best available clinical research evidence into practice is a complex process that requires significant time and effort. Clinicians rarely have the time required to sift through and evaluate copious amounts of literature to determine the best clinical decision for each patient encounter in a clinical setting. Information technology helps to streamline this process by enabling us to easily access, analyze, evaluate, and disseminate vast amounts of information, including clinical research and evidence-based practice guidelines. But in fast-paced clinical settings, decisions must be made quickly and having access to best practice recommendations is critical. Health information technologies such as electronic health records (EHRs), clinical decision support systems (CDSSs), and wireless and handheld devices are essential tools for integrating research evidence into practice. When evidence-based protocols are integrated into health information technology, the system can then be used by the provider or nurse to guide clinical decision making for an individual patient at the point of care. CDSS is an example of an information technology tool that is designed for that purpose.

CDSSs analyze computer-based EHR data to assist healthcare providers to follow evidence-based clinical guidelines at the point of care through digital prompts and reminders. Research shows that CDSS is effective, leads to improvements in quality of care, and has the potential to reduce disparities in care (Centers for Disease Control and Prevention [CDC], 2021). The primary purpose of clinical decision support (CDS) is to provide timely information that will assist clinicians, patients, and other members of the healthcare team in making informed healthcare decisions. Examples of CDS include order sets to treat a specific condition, recommendations relevant to the patient situation, preventive care reminders, and alerts to prevent adverse events or potentially dangerous clinical decisions. CDS can be implemented and accessed on the Internet, personal computers, EHR networks, handheld devices, and paper-based systems (Agency for Healthcare Research and Quality [AHRQ], 2019). According to HealthIT.gov (2018), important benefits of CDS include:

- Increased quality of care and enhanced outcomes.
- Avoidance of errors and adverse events.
- Improved efficiency, cost effectiveness, and satisfaction for provider and patient.

CDS must be well-designed and strategically placed in the clinical and EHR workflow to ensure informed decisions can be made quickly and be acted upon (2018).

The precursor to CDS as a technology tool in EHRs is paper-based clinical practice guidelines (CPG) which were developed to help practitioners and

1 Thank you to Joyce Brettner, DNP, MAHS, RN-BC for contributing her expertise and knowledge for this section.

patients to make informed healthcare decisions. With the increased adoption of EHRs, CDS aimed to maximize technology to enhance a clinician's ability to make evidence-informed decisions by presenting recommendations electronically that are based on the best available scientific evidence and the patient situation. CDS is not intended to replace the clinician's clinical judgment, patient preference, or the patient's unique care needs (Tcheng et al., 2017). Ideally, the EHR supports the triggering of a care plan or order set from assessment data, interdisciplinary problem lists, and medical diagnoses at appropriate points across the care continuum. Importantly, the care plans and order sets, when used in the care of an individual patient, require the clinical judgment of the care provider to individualize the standard plan or order set to the unique needs of the specific patient. Decision support systems provide hyperlinks to the evidence summaries or guidelines on which the vendor plan of care or standard order set is based and support links to relevant organizational policies, quality measures, and resources.

Decision support can be provided apart from the electronic health record. Vendors offer searchable libraries of evidence-based summaries on clinical topics. The summaries may include nursing care plans, recommendations from national guidelines, and quality measures. Patient teaching handouts, procedure videos, and links to external sources are often included in these products. Linked referential CDS is information the clinician accesses via a hyperlink. According to the CMS, linked referential CDS provides the user diagnostic and therapeutic reference information that aligns with standards and specifications (CMS, 2017). It is also called *pull* guidance because it requires providers to interrupt their workflow and seek information. In contrast, clinical guidance embedded in an EHR is referred to as *push* guidance because it is provided to the clinician without any effort on their part. Generally, the availability of referential information is thought to have less impact on care planning and decision making than actionable information.

Present and Future

Most assuredly, access to research evidence and evidence-based practice recommendations have greatly improved in recent years; the formats are more clinician friendly and professional associations are promoting awareness of evidence-based practices at conferences, on their websites, and in journals. Proprietary products are being upgraded; government and privately funded initiatives in many countries are promoting evidence-based practice and funding studies about how to translate research findings into practice. Thus, progress in moving research evidence into practice has improved but is still a work in progress (Dang et al., 2022).

Wrap-Up

At this point, we suggest you pause to consider all that has been presented to this point in this book. **Figure 17-2** portrays the really big picture beginning with recognition that knowledge for a particular issue of practice is lacking, proceeding through the steps of knowledge production and EBP and finally achieving best practice. It is a long path, but we owe it to our patients, to society, to our profession, and to ourselves as professional nurses to walk the EBP walk.

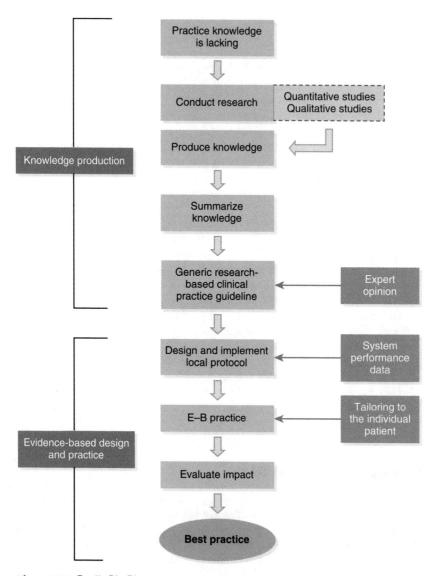

Figure 17-2 Really Big Picture

References

Agency for Healthcare Research and Quality. (2019, June). *Clinical decision support.* https://www
.ahrq.gov/cpi/about/otherwebsites/clinical-decision-support/index.html
Berwick, D. M., Nolan, T. W., & Whittington, J. (2008). The triple aim: care, health, and cost.
Health Affairs, 27(3), 759–769. https://doi.org/10.1377/hlthaff.27.3.759
Centers for Disease Control and Prevention. (2021, July 22). *Implementing clinical decision support
systems.* https://www.cdc.gov/dhdsp/pubs/guides/best-practices/clinical-decision-support.htm

Centers for Medicare and Medicaid Services. (2017, August). *Eligible professional Medicaid EHR incentive program stage 3 objectives and measures objective 3 of 8.* https://www.cms.gov/Regulations-and-Guidance/Legislation/EHRIncentivePrograms/Downloads/MedicaidEPStage3_Obj3.pdf

Centers for Medicare & Medicaid Services. (2021, December 1). *Quality measurement and quality improvement.* https://www.cms.gov/Medicare/Quality-Initiatives-Patient-Assessment-Instruments/MMS/Quality-Measure-and-Quality-Improvement-

Centers for Medicare and Medicaid Services. (2022, October 7). *Hospital quality initiative.* http://www.cms.gov/Medicare/Quality-Initiatives-Patient-Assessment-Instruments/HospitalQualityInits/index.html?redirect=/HospitalQualityInits/

Dang, D., Dearholt, S., Bissett, K., Ascenzi, J., & Whalen, M. (2022). *Johns Hopkins evidence-based practice for nurses and healthcare professionals: Model and guidelines* (4th ed.). Sigma Theta Tau International.

Dearing, J.W. (2009). Applying diffusion of innovation theory to intervention development. *Research on Social Work Practice, 19*(5), 503–518. https://doi.org/10.1177/1049731509335569

Drucker, P. F. (2002). *The discipline of innovation.* Harvard Business Review. https://hbr.org/2002/08/the-discipline-of-innovation

Eisenberg, J. M., Foster, N. E., Meyer, G., & Holland, H. (2001). Federal efforts to improve quality of care: The Quality Interagency Coordination Task Force (QuIC). *The Joint Commission Journal on Quality Improvement, 27*(2), 93–100. https://doi.org/10.1016/S1070-3241(01)27009-6

Gray J. R., Grove, S. K., & Sutherland, S. (2017). *Burns and Grove's the practice of nursing research: Appraisal, synthesis, and generation of evidence* (8th ed.). Saunders Elsevier.

Harrison, M. B., Graham, I. D., van den Hoek, J., Dogherty, E. J., Carley, M. E., & Angus, V. (2013). Guideline adaptation and implementation planning: A prospective observational study. *Implementation Science, 8,* Article 49.

Harvey, G., & Kitson, A. (2016). PARIHS revisited: From heuristic to integrated framework for successful implementation of knowledge into practice. *Implementation Science, 11,* Article 33. https://doi.org/10.1186/s13012-016-0398-2

HealthIT.gov. (2018, April 10). *Clinical decision support.* https://www.healthit.gov/topic/safety/clinical-decision-support

Health Resources and Services Administration. (2022). *Clinical quality improvement.* https://bphc.hrsa.gov/technical-assistance/clinical-quality-improvement

Institute for Healthcare Improvement. (2015). *What is a bundle?* http://www.ihi.org/resources/Pages/ImprovementStories/WhatIsaBundle.aspx

Institute of Medicine (US) Committee on Quality of Health Care in America. (2001). *Crossing the Quality chasm: A new health system for the 21st century.* National Academies Press. https://doi.org/10.17226/10027

Iowa Model Collaborative. (2017). Iowa model of evidence-based practice: Revisions and validation. *Worldviews on Evidence-Based Nursing, 14*(3), 175–182. https://doi.org/10.1111/wvn.12223

Jablonski, A. M., DuPen, A. R., & Ersek, M. (2011). The use of algorithms in assessing and managing persistent pain in older adults. *AJN, American Journal of Nursing, 111*(3), 34–43.

Kohn, L. T., Corrigan, J. M., & Donaldson, M. S. (Eds.). (2000). *To err is human: Building a safer health system.* National Academies Press. https://doi.org/10.17226/9728

Lawal, A. K., Rotter, T., Kinsman, L., Machotta, A. K., Ronellenfitsch, U., Scott, S., Goodridge, D., & Plishka, C. (2016). What is a clinical pathway? Refinement of an operational definition to identify clinical pathway studies for a Cochrane systematic review. *BMC Medicine, 14,* Article 35.

Marra, A., Ely, E. W., Pandharipande, P. P., & Patel, M. B. (2017). The ABCDEF bundle in critical care. *Critical Care Clinics, 33*(2), 225–243. https://doi.org/10.1016/j.ccc.2016.12.005

Melnyk, B. M., & Fineout-Overholt, E. (2019). *Evidence-based practice in nursing and healthcare: A guide to best practice* (4th ed.). Wolters Kluwer.

Tcheng, J. E., Bakken, S., Bates, D. W., Bonner, H., Gamdhi, T. K., Josephs, M., Kawamoto, K., Lomotan, E. A., Mackay, E., Middleton, B., Teich, J. M., Weingarten, S., & Lopez, M. H. Eds.). (2017). *Optimizing strategies for clinical decision support: Summary of a meeting series.* National Academy of Medicine. https://nam.edu/optimizing-strategies-clinical-decision-support/

Titler, M. (2018). Translation research in practice: An introduction. *OJIN: The Online Journal of Issues in Nursing, 23*(2). https://doi.org/10.3912/OJIN.Vol32No02Man01

Weberg, D., & Davidson, S. (2019). *Leadership for evidence-based innovation in nursing and health professions* (2nd ed.). Jones & Bartlett.

CHAPTER 18

Evidence-Based Practice Participation

There are several scenarios in which you might get involved in an evidence-based practice (EBP) project. The first would be as a student; then, other opportunities could arise in your work setting—present or future. We thought we could provide a bit of guidance in this regard. Six scenarios will be described, and suggestions will be made regarding each:

1. You decide to do your capstone project around some aspect of evidence-based practice.
2. As a participant in a patient care planning conference, you present research evidence relevant to the care of a patient with a complex issue.
3. As a member of a project team in your work setting, you could be asked to appraise one or several pieces of research evidence and give a short oral presentation about it.
4. You decide to submit an evidence-based poster to be displayed at a congress or conference.
5. You want to present an evidence-based clinical idea or concern to your nurse leader, clinical nurse specialist, or nurse manager.
6. Evidence-based practice really interests you, and you want to further develop your EBP knowledge and skills.

Capstone Project

A capstone project, by definition, requires you to use and connect what you have learned throughout your nursing program. A capstone project focused on evidence-based practice could require you to do some scholarly work but also some work in the clinical setting where you envision an evidence-based change in practice. Your project could follow the Johns Hopkins Nursing Evidence-Based Practice model described in Chapter 17 of this text (Dang et al., 2022). Using this model might require adaptation to the requirements of your program, but it offers a great starting point. Alternatively, if you are currently working in a setting and knowledge of an issue and a credible evidence-based clinical practice guideline that you think should be implemented, your project could start by working with a nurse manager and others to develop an implementation and evaluation plan rather than having to start all the way at the beginning.

Contribute to a Patient Care Conference

When a patient's care presents difficult problems or requires complex discharge arrangements, a patient care planning conference will often be called. The goal of such a conference is to bring together all the people involved in the patient's care to address a particular problem and come up with an approach to the problematic issue or issues. These planning sessions design more effective strategies when someone is assigned to spend an hour looking for research evidence relative to a key issue or issues in the management of the patient's problems. Perhaps there is an evidence-based guideline that is relevant to the patient's sleeping problem. Maybe a systematic review that addresses the issue of whether a teenager can take a shower even though he has external skeletal pins in place can be identified. Increasingly, evidence-based information is being brought to the table at patient care planning conferences.

If a conference is called and you will be involved, you should give some thought to the problems or issues that may be, or should be, discussed. There may be one or two issues for which it would be helpful for all participants to understand effective approaches that are supported by research evidence. If the person who leads the conference does not assign anyone to look at the research evidence about the problem, you might lead the way by doing so.

At the conference, you could bring what you found in your brief search to the table—not in a lecturing way, but in a contributing way. In that regard, we warn against the overused and vague phrase, "research shows." Instead, say something specific like, "I found one systematic review that looked at five studies about sleeping problems in hospitalized adolescents. The reviewers reached the conclusion that. . . ." Have the article with you so anyone who chooses to can look at it. The inclusion of research-based information into the discussion will most likely be valued and will serve to take the exchange beyond opinions to more objective knowledge as the basis for care planning.

Join a Project Team

Another alternative is for those already working as nurses or health care providers in a health system. For instance, if your unit is looking at its use of special beds and bed surfaces for patients at risk of skin breakdown, you might suggest the initiation of a work group to develop a decision algorithm or decision tree regarding the use of special beds and surfaces. Working together using steps 1–12 of the Johns Hopkins model, the team could then bring their findings to a unit meeting to get support for moving forward with designing an action plan.

You could organize your talk in the following way:

- Give a summary of the systematic review along the same lines as the information in the synopsis part of the systematic review appraisal guide.
- State your overall impression of the credibility of the conclusions along with your reasons for confidence or concerns.

- State your opinion regarding the clinical significance of the conclusions.
- Address the applicability of the findings and conclusions to the patients seen on your unit and the resources that will be available.

Make a Poster

Professional conferences and congresses often issue calls for oral presentations or posters of research studies and EBP projects. A summary of evidence regarding a clinical question often makes a relevant and interesting poster. Posters are usually mounted on boards in specified areas at congresses, and people walk around and read them. Most congresses require that a person be present with the poster at specified times so people can ask questions.

Let's say that the bed surface-skin breakdown group's work from your unit is moving along well, and you notice a call from the National Association of Orthopaedic Nurses (NAON) for posters at its spring congress. Because your workgroup has not finished its work on the algorithm/protocol, you decide to submit a poster regarding just the evidence used to produce the algorithm. Most associations allow the submission of work-in-progress posters. You would first submit to NAON an abstract of your poster's content. Then, if it is accepted, you would proceed to create the poster using PowerPoint or similar presentation software and produce it using a poster-making machine.

When making a poster, you have to be very selective about the information included. If it has too much information or if the information is presented in a disorganized way, people will avoid stopping to read it or will read part of it and walk away. The idea of a poster is to present the main ideas—it is like an abstract. If the person looking at the poster is interested in knowing more, they will ask you some questions. You (the person explaining the poster) are the real resource; the poster is mostly just a lure.

There are no ironclad rules for how to design a poster, but a few suggestions may help. In regard to the design of the poster, information should be grouped in some logical way with a header for each block and three to five points under each header. You might want to have a list of the EbCPGs and systematic reviews that are referenced in the poster for people who ask for them, or you could have interested persons write down their email address, and after the congress, you can send a list of references to them.

There are multiple research poster templates out there. A quick Google search will show you a variety of examples to match both your project and your budget. Having a poster at a congress is a fun and informative experience. A lot of people will talk with you, and you will learn a lot. It's definitely a recommended step in your professional growth and development.

Present an Idea or Concern

Now let's say that while you were at the congress, you went to a session about preventing and managing confusion in elderly patients with hip fractures. You went to the session because this issue has recently been a challenge in caring for several patients on your unit. You decide to see what research evidence is available on the topic and to talk with the clinical nurse specialist for your unit. A 15-minute search on CINAHL—using the terms *delirium, hip fracture*, and *interventions*, with the *research only* and *evidence-based practice* filters on—turns up two EbCPGs, an systematic review, and several research articles about preventing and managing delirium in patients with hip fracture; they indicate that pain relief is clearly important.

To talk to the clinical nurse specialist or nurse leader, it is best to make an appointment. Catch-as-catch-can in the hallway usually does not work; interruptions are bound to occur, or you may catch them when they have something else on their mind. Here are some suggestions for preparing for your appointment:

- Be able to give some recent examples of why you think delirium prevention and management is a problem on your unit. Specific patient examples would support your claim that delirium care is not as good as it could be.
- Briefly describe the research evidence you found on your quick search. It might be good to give them a copy of several of the research abstracts or URLs you found.
- If your unit already has a protocol about this topic, look at it before your appointment. If the protocol is evidence-based and well written, maybe the appropriate action would be to bring it anew to the staff's attention along with any new research. If the protocol is not helpful, up to date, or consistent with newer research, point out its shortcomings.
- Ask their opinion about how to get things moving to make a change, but have an idea or two in mind beforehand.

There is no guarantee you will get a positive response and good follow-through, but the chances are good, and the cause is a good one.

Build Your EBP Knowledge and Skills

If the transfer of scientific knowledge into practice really interests you, you should consider developing your EBP skills beyond what you have learned in the course you are now taking. You could take additional coursework or continuing education about EBP. Some clinical congresses offer EBP pre-congress sessions or multiday EBP workshops. Alternatively, you might ask your nurse manager to give you paid time to attend an in-depth EBP workshop. Several of the most well-known EBP models offer these types of workshops, including Johns Hopkins. The active learning that occurs in these kinds of programs will prepare you to fully participate in—even lead—EBP projects in your clinical unit or agency. Another option would be that when seeking employment at a large medical center, ask about in-house EBP training. Quite a few medical centers have them. In summary, there are numerous ways to be involved in evidence-based practice and thereby contribute to good patient care and professional exchange.

Reference

Dang, D., Dearholt, S., Bissett, K., Ascenzi, J., & Whalen, M. (2022). *Johns Hopkins evidence-based practice for nurses and healthcare professionals: Model and guidelines* (4th ed.). Sigma Theta Tau International.

CHAPTER 19

Point-of-Care Adaptations

Evidence-based care protocols help incorporate scientifically supported care actions into care planning and promote consistency of care. However, as noted earlier, most scientific evidence is largely based on what works best *on average*. Thus, even when the research evidence is strong in support of a care approach for a specified patient group, we cannot expect everyone in that group to benefit from it. Additionally, even if it is clinically effective, the care approach may not be acceptable to all persons. For these reasons, nurses should enter into an exchange with each patient during care planning and care delivery to determine if the care being given is accomplishing what it should and to learn what they want from care. When care is adapted or modified to individual responses and preferences, it is considered individualized, person-centered, or tailored to the individual. To achieve individualized care the nurse must:

- Truly be present to the patient when in their presence.
- Be attuned to the patient's problems, complaints, preferences, values, goals, and beliefs.
- Share decision making about care.

Individualized Care Story

A nurse saw a patient in a diabetes mellitus clinic. Listening to their chest, the nurse heard mild wheezes and looked into their healthcare record to determine how their asthma was being managed. The patient was prescribed a PRN bronchodilator delivered via inhaler with a spacer for relief of shortness of breath and a steroid inhaler with a spacer once a day. The nurse asked the patient how often they used the inhalers. They said they used the PRN bronchodilator 4 to 6 times a day but did not use the steroid inhaler very often because "it has a bad taste, it dries out my mouth, and it ruins the taste of good food." They said they would rather use the PRN inhaler. The nurse explained the value of the steroid medication in preventing asthma symptoms and why it should be taken regularly. The patient said, "Yeah, I know."

The nurse then asked to see the patient's PRN inhaler, which they had with them, and noticed that the patient was not using the spacer. The patient said they didn't use the spacer with the inhaler because it didn't fit in their shirt pocket. The nurse asked whether they used the spacer on their steroid inhaler—No. The nurse suggested that they use the spacer with the steroid inhaler as it would get the medication deeper into their airway and not so much in their mouth. The nurse also suggested gargling with warm water and brushing their teeth after using the steroid inhaler. Lastly, the nurse suggested that the patient could continue using the PRN inhaler without a spacer and they would see how that went. The patient seemed agreeable to that so the nurse showed the patient how to use the spacer and gave them a pamphlet to refer to if they had questions about its use when they returned home.

At the patient's next visit a month later, the patient said they were using the steroid inhaler with the spacer every morning before they brushed their teeth and that the mouth problem was *okay*. The patient also thought that they were using the PRN inhaler less often. The patient had no wheezing at the time of this visit.

This is individualized care. The nurse recognized the importance of the steroid inhaler as part of the asthma management protocol, but at the same time was attuned to the patient's complaint about its oral effects. The nurse asked the right questions to get at how the patient was using their inhalers and together they came up with an approach that was both effective and acceptable to the patient.

At the point of care, the clinician and patient together decide if an evidence-based protocol endorsed by the agency or health system is acceptable and effective. The patient brings to this discussion responses to treatments, preferences, experiences, life goals, family support, and resources. The clinician brings clinical knowledge, prior experience with similar cases, interpersonal sensitivity, information about the patient's clinical condition, and professional judgment. Through such an exchange, evidence-based protocols are tailored to the individual patient (Engle et al., 2021).

Standardized protocols only go so far in specifying how care should be given. There still will be situations for which there is not an applicable protocol or when the protocol does not address a specific issue relating to the protocol. As a nurse committed to evidence-based practice you should think: *I wonder if there is any research evidence about this to guide what I do.* However, clearly, you only have a limited amount of time in which to get an answer to your question. The rest of this chapter is about websites or apps that can be accessed with handheld e-devices. Importantly, many of these resources provide short-form summaries in everyday language. In some cases, the evidence has even been appraised, and an overall statement of its quality included in the summary or for each recommendation.

Point-of-Care Evidence-Based Practice Story

A home health nurse was caring for two older persons with chronic lower leg ulcers. One was a 92-year-old patient whose wound was shallow, just lightly exuding, and periodically had a small amount of necrotic tissue. Compression stockings had been tried but were not tolerated by the patient, so just leg elevation and ACE elastic bandages were used. The dressing was being changed daily and the wound was cleansed with sterile water; a 21-day treatment with an enzymatic debriding agent had removed necrotic tissue. The nurse went to the National Guideline Clearinghouse, the Registered Nurses' Association of Ontario, and the Cochrane Collaboration websites to search for clinical practice guidelines and systematic reviews.

The nurse had heard about several medications that might promote healing. The nurse searched the databases using the terms *leg ulcer* or *venous leg ulcers*. Among the helpful documents were three guidelines and several systematic reviews about the management of open wounds in patients with lower extremity venous disease.

From these, the nurse had several evidence-based ideas for promoting the healing of this patient's leg ulcer, including recommending walking in place and/or calf muscle pumping every 2 hours to increase circulation. The nurse also learned that leg elevation is most effective when the feet are above the level of the heart (e.g., putting the foot of the bed on blocks or placing a wedge under the foot end of the mattress). The strong research support for the effectiveness of compression therapy convinced the nurse that they should reconsider compression alternatives to see if they could find one that the patient would tolerate and found several alternative products. In the end, the nurse spent a little over an hour and learned about some interventions they hadn't tried that have research support and confirmed the strong support for compression therapy as the mainstay of treatment.

From Mobile Devices

Okay, so maybe you don't have an hour and need some information quicker. First a caveat: there are hundreds of healthcare and nursing sites and resources available for various clinical specialities areas and purposes, but they are not all evidence based. Some are designed to provide reference information such as normal lab values, drug interactions, medical diagnosis signs and symptoms, or drug calculation. If you are looking for evidence-based information to guide you in giving care, you should rely on the sites of recognized organizations and associations that inform users about how they produce their care guidance or systematic research reviews.

Getting evidence-based information doesn't have to involve an extensive search every time. In fact, many healthcare systems already have resources available to you. If they don't or if they don't have ones that you feel get to the question you are asking, you may find it helpful to put together a list of bookmarks that make available evidence-based guidelines or systematic reviews in your area of practice. You may also mark a few sites of organizations that produce EbCPGs and systematic reviews quite broadly that you can check out when you encounter clinical issues outside your usual area of practice. The time spent compiling such a list could save you a lot of time later on and help you avoid having to do online searches using a general browser that brings up all kinds of commercial sites.

The websites and apps listed below should help you in starting your list of online resources. All are sites providing evidence-based care information in formats suitable for access from mobile devices. Some cover many areas of practice, whereas others are specific to a particular area of practice. Some include summarized forms of full guidelines or systematic reviews; others just access them in full. Some are free, and some charge. Most are available for iPad/iPhone and Android devices. The information provided in the following sections is taken from the websites listed.

PubMed

PubMed databases can be searched for citations using *PubMed Mobile*. The site uses keyword search but also uses filters for article type, which makes it easy to zero in on systematic reviews. Questions can be asked in the PICOT format, and there are links to full-text articles. It is available through multiple interfaces and in multiple languages.

- http://www.ncbi.nlm.nih.gov/m/pubmed/

National Guideline Clearinghouse

The National Guideline Clearinghouse guideline summaries are available in HTML format and downloadable to mobile devices—just click the HTML link at the top of any summary page.

- http://www.guideline.gov/resources/mobile-resources.aspx

U.S. Preventive Services Task Force

The Electronic Preventive Services Selector (ePSS) is designed to help primary care clinicians and healthcare teams make timely decisions regarding appropriate screening, counseling, and preventive services for their patients. The ePSS is available both as a web application and a mobile application. The ePSS information is based on the current, evidence-based recommendations of the U.S. Preventive Services Task Force and can be searched by specific patient characteristics, such as age, sex, and selected behavioral risk factors.

- http://epss.ahrq.gov/PDA/index.jsp

Canadian Task Force on Preventive Health Care

The Canadian Task Force on Preventive Health Care (CTFPHC) mobile app helps primary care practitioners rapidly access CTFPHC guidelines and resources at the point of care and while on the go. The app contains guideline and recommendation summaries, knowledge translation tools, and links to additional resources.

- http://canadiantaskforce.ca/resources/ctfphc-mobile-app/

Professional Associations

Many professional associations offer apps that access evidence-based guidelines and other information related to their specialities. Here are just a few examples. This list is not exhaustive and new ones are routinely becoming available.

Registered Nurses' Association of Ontario

Condensed versions of a wide range of nursing best practice guidelines are available via its PBG app or via a web version. Their guidelines are available in English and French.

- http://rnao.ca/bpg/pda
- http://pda.rnao.ca

Wound Ostomy and Continence Nurses Society

The app provides access to guidelines for prevention and management of pressure ulcers, management of the patient with a fecal ostomy, management of wounds in patients with lower extremity arterial disease, management of wounds in patients with lower extremity neuropathic disease, and management of wounds in patients with lower extremity venous disease.

- http://www.wocn.org/?page=guidelinesapp

National Association of Nurse Practitioners in Women's Health Oncology

This association offers a free app intended to be a convenient quick reference during a well-woman visit. It consists of the most commonly used clinical guidelines, and the recommendations are age based.

- https://www.npwh.org/pages/mobile-app

Association of Operating Room Nurses

The Association of Operating Room Nurses offers an ebook mobile app featuring e-b guidelines for perioperative practice. It is available for purchase via computer, smartphones, and tablets.

- http://www.aorn.org/aorn-org/guidelines/purchase-guidelines/ebook -mobile-app

Infectious Diseases Society of America

The Guideline Central app offers mobile versions of summarized Infectious Diseases Society of America's guidelines. This interactive app features keyword search of pocket cards and quick reference tools even when Internet access and cellular service are not available.

- http://www.idsociety.org/guidelinesapp/

Hartford Institute for Geriatric Nursing

The ConsultGeriRN feature aims to help professionals make care decisions right from the bedside. The information is based on the most current evidence-based practice standards; topics include delirium, agitation, confusion, and fall prevention. The app is available through iTunes.

- https://itunes.apple.com/us/app/consultgerirn/id5783601

American College of Physicians

The American College of Physicians' high-quality guidelines are available via a mobile app. Guidelines are in an easy-to-read, interactive format.

- https://itunes.apple.com/us/app/acp-clinical-guidelines/id618318388?mt=8
- https://play.google.com/store/apps/details?id=com.ACP.ClinicalGuidelines

Companies

The companies that produce clinical reference sources for mobile devices often include evidence-based information in the form of care sheets, care plans, monographs, and hyperlinks to research evidence. Several are designed specifically for nurses and others are interdisciplinary.

Our Ending—Your Beginning

Evidence-based practice is not a window dressing on *professional* nursing practice— it's an integral component of it. Reading research articles and evidence-based practice guidelines, appraising them, and deciding whether to change practice based on them comprise a professional skill set. Like all new skills, there is a learning curve, but if you have paid attention and you remember to use the resources available to you, the steepest part of the curve will be behind you. Like all skills, it requires some maintenance to keep the skill set sharp and current. Fortunately, a small amount of effort will benefit patients and make your professional dialogue and career more intellectually interesting and rewarding. That's enough for now; you've got this. Go out and do great things!

References

Engle, R. L., Mohr, D. C., Holmes, S. K., Seibert, M. N., Afable, M., Leyson, J., & Meterko, M. (2021). Evidence-based practice and patient-centered care: Doing both well. *Health Care Management Review*, 46(3), 174–184. https://doi.org/10.1097/HMR.0000000000000254

Glossary

A

Absolute benefit increase The difference between the percentage of persons in one treatment group who attained a clinical milestone and the percentage of persons in another treatment group who attained it.

Across-studies analysis Comparison, contrast, and pattern searching in findings from two or more studies; the analysis examines the studies as a body of evidence.

Algorithm A step-by-step instruction for solving a clinical problem; often consists of a series of yes/no questions leading to one of several possible decisions or actions.

Applicability The relevance of research evidence to a particular setting considering the similarity of the setting's patients to those in the studies, as well as the safety, feasibility, and expected benefit of implementing the findings.

Appraisal Making objective, systematic judgments regarding the credibility, clinical significance, and applicability of research evidence to determine if changes in practice should be made based on the evidence.

B

Bias A study influence or action (such as preconceptions or research methods) that produces distorted results, i.e., results that deviate from actuality. The most common sources of research methods bias are design bias, selection bias, measurement bias, and procedural bias.

Blinding Steps taken in experimental studies to keep study staff and participants from knowing which treatment group a person is in; the function of blinding is to prevent personal predilections from influencing responses to the treatment or rating of responses.

Bonferroni correction A lowering of the level at which a p-value is considered significant; it is used to prevent a type 1 conclusion error resulting from multiple tests on the same data.

C

Care bundle A group of evidence-based interventions related to a health condition that, when executed together, result in better outcomes than when implemented individually.

Care design The process of using knowledge, information, and data to develop a plan of care for a patient population or for an individual patient.

Case-control study A study in which patients who have an outcome of interest and similar patients who do not have the outcome are identified; then, the researcher looks back to determine exposures and experiences that could have contributed to the outcome occurring or not occurring.

Chance difference A difference in outcomes of a study that occurred in the sample of the study but would probably not be found in the target population. It is inferred from a non-significant statistical result (that is, a data-based p-value greater than the specified decision point p-level).

Chance variation The variability in sample averages that is expected whenever one measures a trait, behavior, physiological state, or outcome in two or more samples from the same population.

Clinical decision support The function of a computerized clinical information system that uses inputted patient data to provide agency protocols, information, and more general knowledge relevant to the care of the patient.

Clinical practice guideline A generic set of recommendations regarding the management of a clinical condition, problem, or situation. Ideally, the guideline is produced by a panel of experts and is based on rigorous analysis of research evidence.

Clinical protocol An agency standard of care that sets forth care that should be given to patients with a specified health condition, treatment, or circumstances. Protocols take a variety of forms including care maps, decision algorithms, standard order sets, clinical procedures, care bundles, and standardized plans of care; they guide care in combination with clinical judgment and patient preference.

Clinical significance In quantitative studies, an appraiser's judgment that a research finding indicates a large enough intervention effect or association between variables to have clinical meaning in terms of patients' health or well-being. In qualitative studies, an appraiser's judgment that the findings are informative and useful. The term can be applied in a more general sense to recommendations of clinical practice guidelines and conclusions of systematic reviews.

Coefficient of determination (r_2) The proportion (or percentage) of a variable that is associated with, or explained by, another variable.

Cohort study A study in which two groups of people are identified, one with an exposure of interest and another without the exposure. The two groups are followed forward to determine if the outcome of interest occurs.

Comparison group In an experimental study, the group that was not given the experimental treatment.

Conclusion error A wrong statistical conclusion reached because of a chance statistical result, a sample size that is too small, large variations in scores, or extraneous variables.

Confidence interval (CI) An extraneous interval that estimates the result that would be found if the whole target population were included in the study; it is an interval around the sample result.

Confounding variable A variable whose presence affects the variables being studied so that the results do not reflect the actual relationship between the variables being studied. It is an uncontrolled or unrecognized extraneous variable that exerted influence on the variables studied.

Consecutive series A method of obtaining a sample in which starting at a certain point, every person who meets the inclusion criteria is asked to participate in the study, and enrollment continues until the predetermined sample size is reached. It is essentially a convenience sample, although it is less prone to bias than the researcher inviting persons to participate based on his own schedule and inclinations.

Control Study methods that (1) decrease, isolate, or eliminate the influence of extraneous variables; (2) prevent bias from influencing the results; and (3) limit the amount of chance variation.

Control group The group given the experimental treatment in an experimental study.

Convenience sample A sample that is drawn from an accessible group of people who the researcher thinks are part of a larger target population.

Correlation A relationship between two interval or rank-order variables in which their values move in accordance with one another to a lesser, moderate, or greater degree.

Correlational research Research in which the relationship between two or more variables is studied without active intervention by the researcher.

Credibility A characteristic conferred on a finding. The judgment that a finding is trustworthy and not determined by bias, error, extraneous variables, or inaccurate interpretation of the data.

D

Database A structured, updated collection of informational records about articles, books, and other resources; access to the records is managed with computer software. Some examples are CINAHL, MEDLINE, and PsycINFO.

Delivery system The context in which direct clinical care is given; it comprises a network of logistics including patient flow, scheduling, communications, supplies and equipment availability, role responsibilities, work patterns, accountability structures, and other work dynamics that support direct patient care.

Dependent variable Also called the outcome variable. In experimental research, the response or outcome that is expected to depend on or be caused

by the independent variable. It occurs later in time than the independent variable.

Descriptive study A quantitative study that aims to portray a naturally occurring situation, event, or response to illness; data consists of counts of how often something occurs and breakdowns of various aspects of the situation into categories or levels.

Dichotomous variable A variable that has only two possible values, for example, readmitted/not readmitted.

E

Effect size A statistical representation of the strength of a relationship between two variables; commonly, the size of an intervention's impact on an outcome variable relative to the impact of the comparison intervention.

Error Distortion of data or results caused by mistakes in sampling or measuring or failure to follow study procedures.

Ethnographic research A qualitative research tradition that examines cultures and subcultures to understand how they work and the meaning of members' behaviors.

Evidence Objective knowledge or information used as the basis for a clinical protocol, clinical decision, or clinical action. Evidence sources include research, agency data regarding system performance and patient outcomes, large healthcare databases, and expert opinion.

Evidence-based clinical practice guideline A set of recommended clinical actions for a clinical problem or population that are based to some degree on research evidence.

Evidence-based practice (EBP) The use of care methods that have been endorsed by an agency because available evidence indicates they are effective.

Experimental group The group in an experimental study that received the treatment of interest, which may be new or not yet definitively tested.

Experimental study A study aimed at comparing the effects of two or more interventions on clinical outcomes. It is characterized by random assignment of participants to treatment groups, careful measurement of outcomes, and control of as many extraneous variables as is feasible to achieve maximum confidence in causal conclusions.

Extraneous variable A variable that is outside the interests of the study but that may influence the data being collected and lead to wrong conclusions. Researchers try to identify them in advance so as to eliminate or control their influence.

F

Findings The interpretation of study results into statements that are slightly more general than the statistical results.

G

Generalizability A judgment about the extent to which the findings of a study will be similar outside the sample in which they were found, i.e., in other practice populations.

Grounded theory methodology A qualitative tradition of inquiry that is conducted to capture social processes that play out in situations of interest; the goal is to incrementally generate a theory that accounts for behavior or decisions.

Guideline A set of recommendations to manage a clinical condition, problem, or situation.

H

Hawthorne effect A change in participants' responses or behaviors because they are aware they are in a study.

Hypothesis A formal statement of the expected results of a study. Hypotheses are tested by data collection and analysis.

I

Impact As used with the evidence-based practice impact model, it is the effect evidence-based practice has on patients' outcomes and experiences of health, illness, and health care.

Independent variable Also called the intervention/treatment variable. In an experimental study, the variable that is manipulated or varied by the researcher to create an effect on the dependent variable. It occurs first in time relative to the dependent variable.

Institutional review board (IRB) An agency or university committee that reviews the design and procedures of studies prior to their being conducted in the care setting. The purpose of the review is to ensure that the research is ethical and that the rights of study participants will not be violated. IRBs are federally regulated.

Instrument Also referred to as a measurement tool. A way of measuring something. The instrument can be a laboratory test, a questionnaire, a rating guide for observations, or a scored assessment form, to name a few.

Integrative research review A type of systematic review in which the findings from various studies are integrated using logical reasoning augmented by findings tables and lists. The goal of an integrative research review is to summarize the research knowledge regarding a topic.

Internal consistency An evaluation of the extent to which the items/questions that compose a measurement instrument capture the underlying concept. A commonly used measure of internal consistency is Cronbach's α.

Interrater reliability The degree to which two or more raters who independently assign a code or score to something assign the same or very similar codes/scores.

Intervention In the research context, intervention is the clinical therapies, action, or courses of action that are evaluated in the study.

L

Level of significance The prespecified decision point for the level of significance or alpha (α). The level of significance is the probability that the event could have occurred by chance. If the level is low, for example 0.05, the probability of that event occurring by chance is small, thus we can say the event is significant.

M

Measurement error The difference in a value obtained by a measurement activity and the actual/true value.

Meta-analysis A systematic research review involving a statistical pooling of the results from several (or many) quantitative studies examining an issue to produce a statistical result with the larger sample size.

Meta-synthesis A systematic research review in which findings from several (or many) qualitative studies examining an issue are merged to produce generalizations and theories.

N

Number needed to treat A representation of treatment effect indicating the number of persons who would need to be treated with the more effective treatment to achieve one additional good outcome (over what would be achieved by using the less effective treatment).

O

Outcome measurement The instrument or tool used to quantify a dependent variable.

Outlier Data contributed by a single study participant that is extreme and considerably outside the range of the other scores in the data set.

P

Phenomenological research A qualitative research tradition used to examine human experiences. The methods seek to understand how the context of the persons' lives affect the meaning they assign to their experiences; the methods rely on inductively building understanding of the experience across several, a few, or a small number of persons.

PICOTS An acronym standing for the elements that should be considered when conducting an evidence-based project and when searching a database for studies. P = population; I = intervention or issue; C = comparison intervention; O = outcome(s); T = timing; S = setting.

p-level The prespecified decision point for the level of significance; databased p-values above this level are considered statistically not significant.

Point-of-care design Care planning for a particular patient that takes place at the bedside or in the patient–nurse encounter; it includes either modification of a protocol or new courses of action not specified by an existing protocol.

Population A group of persons or entities with an important characteristic or characteristics in common.

Power analysis A way of determining sample size that factors in the size of the difference or association expected, the *p*-value cut point, and the probability of finding a difference or relationship that exists.

Projected population Based on the profile of a sample, the population to which the results of a study are believed to apply.

Protocol A clinical protocol is an agency standard of care that sets forth care that should be given to patients with a specified health condition, treatment, or circumstances. Protocols take a variety of forms including care maps, decision algorithms, standard order sets, clinical procedures, care bundles, and standardized plans of care; they guide care in combination with clinical judgment and patient preference.

***p*-value** The data-based probability that the obtained result is attributable to chance variation. This probability is compared to a previously chosen level of significance *p*-level to reach a conclusion about whether the relationship or difference found is statistically significant, i.e., likely to exist in the target population.

Q

Qualitative content analysis A group of data analysis techniques used by qualitative researchers to derive meaning from the content of textual data. It typically involves developing a series of codes from the data.

Qualitative description A qualitative research method that produces straightforward descriptions of participants' experiences in language as similar to the participants' native language as possible.

Qualitative research Inquiry regarding human phenomena that refrains from imposing assumptions on study participants and situations. Its purposes include exploration, description, and theory generation.

Quality filter An assessment of the methodological quality of studies using explicit criteria; it is used in conducting systematic reviews to separate studies of different methodological soundness or to eliminate poorly conducted studies.

Quality improvement An agency's programs aimed at improving the safety, timeliness, patient-centeredness, and efficiency of care delivery systems.

Quantitative research Inquiry that (1) examines preidentified issues; (2) uses designs that control extraneous variables; (3) uses numeric measures to determine levels of various variables; and (4) analyzes data using statistical or graphing methods.

Quasi-experimental A type of intervention research in which either random assignment to control groups or control over the intervention and setting is not possible.

R

Random assignment A chance-based procedure used to assign study participants to a treatment or comparison group. Each participant has an equal chance of being assigned to either treatment group. It serves to distribute participant characteristics evenly in both groups.

Randomized clinical trial (RCT) An experimental study that involves advanced testing of an intervention using defined study protocols typically with a large, diverse sample.

Random sample A sample created by one of several methods by which every person in the population has a greater than zero chance of being included in the sample.

Relationship In research, a connection between two variables in which one influences the other, both influence each other, or both are influenced by a third variable.

Reliability The degree to which a measuring instrument consistently obtains the same or similar measurement values.

Research design A framework or general guide regarding how to structure studies conducted to answer a certain type of research question.

Research evidence Findings of individual studies, conclusions of systematic reviews of research, and research-based recommendations of soundly produced clinical practice guidelines.

Results The outcomes of the numerical and statistical analysis of raw data.

Rigor A quality of a research study that reflects its adherence to recognized standards for its type of study.

S

Sample Persons chosen from a target population to participate in a study. The ideal sample is representative of the target population.

Scope The range or breadth of a question, project, review, or guideline, including a description of what is included.

Search In the context of evidence-based practice, a pursuit to identify all research conducted relevant to a topic. More particularly, the use of a computer search engine to comb through bibliographic databases and other indexes to identify relevant research articles.

Simple random sample A sample that is randomly selected from a list of population members.

Statistical significance A statistical conclusion that a difference or association would likely be found in the population. It is based on a low probability of the result being just due to chance variation.

Study plan A term used in quantitative research to describe how the study will be conducted, including how the sample will be obtained; how the data will be measured, collected, and analyzed; and any control that will be used.

Systematic review A comprehensive and systematic identification, analysis, and summary of research evidence related to a specified issue. A systematic review can use statistics, tabulation, compare-and-contrast methods, or pattern identification to reach conclusions based on the body of studies in the review.

T

Target population The entire group of individuals or organizations to which the sample results are considered applicable. It may be the entire population from which the sample was randomly drawn or a projected population based on a convenience sample's profile.

Test-retest reliability A way of evaluating the consistency with which persons score themselves similarly on the questionnaire at two completions of the questionnaire separated by an appropriate period of time.

Theory Assumptions, concepts, definitions, and/or propositions that provide a cohesive (although tentative) explanation of how a phenomenon is thought to work.

Translational research Also called implementation research. The field of study that investigates how research evidence can effectively be integrated into agency and individual practice.

Treatment In the research context, clinical interventions, therapies, action, or courses of action that are evaluated in the study. The treatment is the independent variable, and its effect on the dependent variables (outcomes) is what is being tested by the study.

True difference A difference found in the study that is large enough that a difference would likely be found in the population; it is inferred from a significant statistical result (that is a data-based p-value less than the specified decision point p-level).

Type 1 conclusion error The conclusion that there is a significant relationship between variables or a significant difference in groups' outcomes when in fact there is not a significant relationship or difference.

Type 2 conclusion error The conclusion that there is not a significant relationship between variables or a significant difference in groups' outcomes when in fact there is a significant relationship or difference.

V

Validity The degree to which a measuring instrument captures the concept it is intended to measure instead of another similar concept.

Variable An attribute of a person, social group, thing, or situation that when measured has two or more categories or possible values.

Index

Page numbers followed by *f*, *t*, and *b* refer to figures, tables, and boxes, respectively.